End Everyday Pain
for **50+**

End Everyday Pain
for 50+

A 10-Minute-a-Day Program of Stretching, Strengthening
and Movement to Break the Grip of Pain

Dr. Joseph Tieri

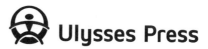 Ulysses Press

To my wife Janice and my daughter Alexis for their love and support,
and to the many patients who entrusted me with their care—thank you.

Published in the United States by
Ulysses Press
P.O. Box 3440
Berkeley, CA 94703
www.ulyssespress.com

ISBN13: 978-1-61243-604-3
Library of Congress Control Number 2016934490

Printed in the United States by United Graphics Inc.

10 9 8 7 6 5 4 3 2 1

Acquisitions editor: Casie Vogel
Managing editor: Claire Chun
Editors: Renee Rutledge and Lily Chou
Proofreader: Lauren Harrison
Indexer: Sayre Van Young
Cover design: what!design @ whatweb.com
Cover artwork: © Jacob Lund/shutterstock.com
Interior design: Jake Flaherty
Production: Caety Klingman, Tainah Harvey
Interior artwork: Rapt Productions except pages 34 (bottom), 37 (top), and 66 © Joseph Tieri and the following artwork from shutterstock.com—pages 19, 28, 39, 42, 43, 62, 70 © Sebastian Kaulitzki; page 20 © Alan Bailey; page 27 © ellepigrafica; page 40 © tsuneomp; page 41 (bottom) © Rawpixel.com; page 47 © ellepigrafica; page 68 © berna namoglu; page 69 © Alila Medical Media; page 71 © BlueRingMedia; page 90 © wavebreakmedia; page 91 Marcin Balcerzak; page 93 © Worachat Limleartworakit; page 95 © solar22; page 96 © Tyler Olson; page 116 © Kinga
Models: Norman Link, Kym Sterner, Joseph Tieri

Distributed by Publishers Group West

Please Note: This book has been written and published strictly for informational purposes, and in no way should be used as a substitute for consultation with health care professionals. You should not consider educational material herein to be the practice of medicine or to replace consultation with a physician or other medical practitioner. The author and publisher are providing you with information in this work so that you can have the knowledge and can choose, at your own risk, to act on that knowledge. The author and publisher also urge all readers to be aware of their health status and to consult health care professionals before beginning any health program.

Contents

Introduction

If you're holding this book in your hands, it's a safe bet that you're experiencing some sort of joint or muscular pain right now, or that you've suffered from it in the recent past. Maybe you're in your 50s or 60s and are beginning to feel some uncomfortable twinges when you spend a few hours in the garden or play a set of tennis. Maybe you've gone beyond twinges and wake up every morning with a stiff neck or a sore back. Maybe you've actually stopped picking up your grandchild because the shoulder pain is too great. Or maybe, like one 54-year-old patient of mine, you feel like you're "living malady to malady" and you're tired of it.

Whatever pain you're experiencing—headaches; neck, shoulder or back pain; hip, knee, or foot pain—this book will help you. I wrote it because I searched for years for a book to recommend to my patients and I couldn't find one that had all the right ingredients. This is not to say that there aren't some good books out there, but I can tell you with certainty that they wouldn't help most of the people that I treat and interact with on a daily basis. My patients are generally busy people who, although dedicated to becoming pain-free, don't have the time or inclination to spend an hour a day doing the numerous routines that typical pain-free books insist on, nor are they all that interested in the detailed anatomy and physiology lessons to which most of these books devote so much attention.

And the pain-free programs failed my patients for another reason, too—even those patients that religiously spent the required time. Most of the books, I discovered, typically advocate one general approach or one solution to fix whatever ails you. The approach might be focused on stretching, or designed around improving posture, or devoted to strengthening weakened muscles. But whatever the focus, any single-pronged approach will fall short. First, when you narrowly focus on one method, devote the necessary time to following its recommendations, and then discover it's not the right approach for you, well, you've spent a lot of time walking (or limping) down the wrong path without seeing any improvement. And second, I don't care how much you stretch, sit upright, or strengthen your back, if you're like my average patient, using just one approach almost certainly will not be enough to get you out of the situation in which you find yourself. Simply stated, to *break the grip* of misalignment and tension on the average adult's body and *end everyday pain*, you need more than one approach or tool—you need some combination of three tools that I've discovered to be essential. As I'll show you later, this is not only more effective, but also saves you time.

But before we talk about the tools—three simple ones—let's talk for a moment about why we need the tools in the first place. As a doctor whose life work is the study and hands-on treatment of the musculoskeletal system (the bones that make up our physical scaffolding, and the joints, muscles, tendons, ligaments, and other soft tissues that support that scaffolding and hold it together), I've had the opportunity to observe and examine literally thousands of bodies over the course of my career. It's not unusual for me to treat a 15-year-old, a 35-year-old, a 55-year-old, and a 75-year-old in a single day. To be able to compare and contrast the bodies of these patients, to not only see but feel the effects of time on the human frame, has been nothing less than revelatory. And what I've seen and felt is that, unless we take preventive measures, our bodies become *gripped* and *molded* into unhealthy positions and patterns as we age, and that these positions and patterns create tension in the body that result in the chronic and recurrent aches and pains, tears and strains, weakness and fatigue, and more serious medical problems that many middle-aged and older people experience on a regular basis.

Advances in Medicine?

Given all of the remarkable advances in medicine we've made over the last 100 years, it may seem odd that we're still so far behind in our ability to properly care for the musculoskeletal system. Actually, it may not be so odd. Many life-saving advances have come about because of our ever-increasing ability to see inside the body using X-rays, MRIs, and other kinds of imaging technology.

Ironically, the indisputable value that these images provide in some cases has created an over-reliance on them in others. While diagnostic films and images are terrific tools for finding disease, they're largely ineffective for addressing musculoskeletal pain and problems.

Likewise with pharmaceutical advances, which offer new hope for many kinds of illness but can only treat or mask the *symptoms* of musculoskeletal problems, not address the problems themselves. Perhaps worse still, when it comes to the human frame, today's technology has distanced modern physicians from the use of their most powerful diagnostic and therapeutic tool—their hands—and has divorced them from the fundamental concepts of prevention and cure.

Your Arthritis Is Not the Problem!

Largely due to this imaging technology, physicians often blame a patient's musculoskeletal aches and pains on arthritis, degenerative changes, bulging and herniated discs, spinal stenosis, and a host of other ills. In truth, as numerous studies have shown (and I'll share these with you in coming chapters), these conditions can be found on the films of many middle-aged and older people, *including those who have no pain!* That's right. There are plenty of people out there with arthritis, bulging discs, and spinal stenosis that have absolutely no pain. It's surprising, isn't it?

So it's not your arthritis, necessarily, that's causing your pain. What's more, most of the typical findings on X-rays and MRIs involving the musculoskeletal system are *symptoms* of a problem and not the problem itself. In other words, your herniated disc isn't the problem—or, at least, it's not the root of the problem—it's a symptom of the problem. And while it may at times be necessary to treat the symptoms, treating a symptom *alone* will never get to the cure.

Avoiding the Premature Breakdown

I believe that we're in the infancy of our understanding of how to properly care for the human musculoskeletal system. If you had lived 150 years ago, it's likely that by the time you reached middle age you'd find it painful to chew, your gums would bleed regularly, and losing a tooth in the middle of a meal would come as no big surprise. It's hard to fathom now, but people didn't realize the essential role of dental hygiene in keeping the teeth and gums healthy. Tooth and gum disease were common early-adulthood phenomena that were accepted as absolutely normal and inevitable.

This seems to me to be an excellent analogy to our current understanding and treatment of the musculoskeletal system. We've come to expect as normal the knee and hip aches, the back and neck stiffness, and the shoulder pain and headaches that so many adults experience. We've come to accept the inevitability of medical intervention of some sort—the use of painkillers, anti-inflammatories, injections, surgical procedures—just to keep pain-free and functioning in our 50s and beyond.

It's my belief that as uneducated as we may be right now when it comes to maintaining the health of our physical frames, there will come a time when we'll look back and see how unnecessary and preventable the premature decline of our musculoskeletal system was—just as we now see so clearly with our teeth. We'll no longer associate the "golden years" with chronic pain and regular visits to the doctor's office. We can and will avoid the premature breakdown of the body's structure and many of the problems that people take for granted as the price of growing older.

How to Use this Book

By utilizing the tools that I teach my patients every day in my office, you, too, will be in a position to easily keep your joints healthy, your muscles happy, and to enjoy a life without pain and unnecessary medical interventions long into your senior years. And the good news is that these quick and easy tools are truly just that: quick and easy. For most of us, they need be no more complicated or time-consuming than the daily care of our teeth. If my suggestions weren't simple to understand and implement, most of my patients wouldn't follow them!

1. **Movement**. Ten minutes a day (or less) of targeted stretching, strengthening, and range-of-motion exercises.

2. **Habit change**. A few habit modifications.

3. **Outside help**. Occasional visits to a hands-on outside practitioner.

And that's it! Revisiting the healthy teeth and gums analogy, it's like advocating that you brush your teeth a couple of times a day, eat a little less sugar, and visit the dentist twice a year. You're welcome to do more if you like (yes, flossing is important, too)—and there's a good chance you'll want to once you see what a difference these simple steps make—but you don't need to.

The ten minutes a day of targeted stretching, strengthening, and range-of-motion (ROM) exercises will help *loosen the grip* of the unhealthy patterns that most of our bodies have adopted in response to our daily work and leisure activities. The habit modifications will *keep your body from slipping back* into those unhealthy patterns. And the visits to an outside practitioner (whether he or she be an osteopath, chiropractor, physical therapist, massage therapist, or other hands-on practitioner—see Chapter Eight, starting on page 98) will *advance your progress* and help you maintain it.

THE THREE ZONES

You've heard it before and it's true: When it comes to the human body, everything is related. The way your head is carried on your body affects your neck, upper back, lower back, pelvis, and on down; the way your feet land on the ground when you walk affects your knees, hips, pelvis, lower back, and on up. When your shoulder really hurts, it's understandable that you want to focus your attention solely on it, but that's not necessarily the wisest choice. Your shoulder is operating in the context of your whole body, especially your whole *upper* body.

Consequently, for the purposes of this book, I've broken the body down into three zones. This allows you to both focus on the painful part and to address the neighboring structures that influence it. **Zone 1** refers to the upper body, including the head, neck, shoulders, and upper back. **Zone 2** is the lower back. **Zone 3** refers to the lower body, including the hips, knees, and feet. And while I hope that you'll read the whole book and follow all of the recommendations in it (no excuses, I've made both the book and the program short), it's fine to focus on the zone that's causing you the most trouble.

Chapter One and Chapter Two discuss how you get to the point of chronic pain and how you can use movement to get out of it.

Chapters Three, Four, and Five cover the different zones of the body: upper body, lower back, and lower body. You don't have to read them in order. Read them according to which zone of the body is causing you the most pain. These chapters contain important information about pain-causing conditions in their respective zones, followed by movement exercises specific to the pertinent area. Start doing the exercises immediately! If you're only working one zone, you'll need *five minutes or less*. If you're working on all three zones, you'll use the Ten-Minute-a-Day Program outlined in Chapter Six.

Chapter Seven quickly identifies some of the pain-causing habits that most of us unconsciously practice.

Chapter Eight offers a deeper understanding of the different kinds of outside practitioners who can support you in breaking the grip and what you can expect when working with the different modalities they employ.

There's plenty of other useful information in the book. Chapter Nine covers the benefits of heat versus ice, rest versus activity, when to wear a brace, important information about treatment reactions, and other pertinent considerations. As I said earlier, I hope you'll want to read about all of the zones and practice all of the exercises because, after all, everything *is* connected. But if you read only the chapters specified above, you'll still have all you need to break the grip and become pain-free. Follow the recommendations and you *will* notice a difference.

Before You Begin

While the vast majority of muscle and joint pain can be alleviated through the program detailed in this book, *you should not be your own doctor when it comes to the actual diagnosis of your pain*. Though it does a poor job of treating and preventing most musculoskeletal issues, modern medicine is very adept at ruling out serious problems. Once tumors, fractures, infections, and unusual medical conditions have been ruled out by your physician and you've decided that you don't want to leap into treating symptoms with prescription drugs, injections, and surgeries, this book can offer you a simple and effective alternative for pain relief that treats the root cause of your problems, not its surface manifestations. At its essence, this book is about the care of the human frame. Many of the greatest minds in medicine and science, from Hippocrates to Thomas Edison, have proclaimed that the human frame, or the physical structure, is the essential foundation for good health, and that the job of the physician is to teach you how to care for it.

And, that being said, let's begin!

CHAPTER ONE
Why Does It Hurt?

Harmony only dwells where obstructions do not exist.

—A. T. Still

The human body is a marvel of architecture and engineering. Nothing has or ever will come close to matching its breathtaking and complex structure and function. Inherent in its design is the remarkable, often unacknowledged ability to recognize problems and to self-correct, an ability that helps us to maintain optimal health. And fortunately for us all, optimal health includes a physical structure that operates smoothly into our middle and later years and wears out gradually and gracefully.

So why, then, do so many middle-aged and older people experience what seems to be a fairly sudden onslaught of aches, pains, and problems that become permanent fixtures in their lives? Why does it suddenly become normal to spend more and more time visiting doctors, taking medications, and contemplating surgeries?

A Sedentary People

For most of human history we've been active people tending to the land, walking to the river for water, and migrating miles at a time to move closer to natural resources and food supplies. And you don't have to go that far back to remember a time when we had to walk to the corner store for milk, hang the laundry on the line to dry, open the garage door manually, and get up from the couch to change the television or radio station. It's actually a relatively recent state of affairs that we live in our homes and work at our jobs with little reason or requirement to actively use our bodies in the normal course of our daily activities.

Though without a doubt modern living has its distinct advantages, some of those advantages come at a price—namely, a body that suffers over time as a result of not moving enough. When I say "enough" here, I mean both in terms of quantity and variety. The body needs both *plenty* of movement and a full *range* of movement to function optimally. We all know that blood needs to circulate throughout our entire body in order to maintain health, and we can understand how activity—movement—promotes this. Movement is also essential to aid in the circulation of lymph, the body's waste disposal fluid. Most pertinent to our specific concern here, though, is the fact that movement promotes the lubrication of joints, and if we fail to get an adequate amount and variety of movement, our joints get stiffer over time and our muscles get tighter and weaker, creating chronic pain and musculoskeletal problems.

Gripped & Molded by Our Habits

Being too sedentary is bad enough, but perhaps the limited and repetitive movements of life in the 21st century cause even more problems. As a result of constantly using our arms out in front of our bodies, as we do when we drive, text, or use a computer, shoulders round and heads move forward; years spent slouching on chairs and couches watching television or reading in bed cause upper and lower backs to round; sitting or lying down with legs or ankles crossed results in legs that turn outward when we walk. In short, over time, our activities and habits grip and mold our bodies in damaging ways.

Unless we're keenly aware of this molding process, it tends to sneak up on us. The human body can take a fair amount of abuse and neglect but, perhaps like the earth itself, sooner or later it reaches a tipping point. The minor aches, pains, and stiffness of middle age can quickly degenerate into the debilitating pain, limited range of motion, and more serious chronic problems of our senior years.

YOU'RE A POSTAL PACKAGE!

Have you ever gone to your mailbox and found an oversized envelope clearly labeled "Do Not Bend" folded and crammed into the box? Was there any doubt in your mind that the contents of the envelope were negatively affected? And how about those family heirlooms from your Great Aunt Mae that arrived in a crushed and dented box marked "Fragile"? Did you shake the box apprehensively, expecting to hear the rattle of fragments of something once whole?

Our bodies can be thought of as envelopes and boxes that contain fragile and valuable contents. When they get "folded" or "dented" through neglect, misuse, or trauma, our contents (not to mention the containers themselves) suffer just like the contents in those damaged envelopes and boxes. The suffering can take many forms, from the more superficial aches and pains in our muscles and joints to the deeper problems of the organs, nerves, and blood vessels. How our bodies get folded and dented and what you can do to fix and prevent this damage is the subject of this book. For now, let's just say that "folded" is a good term to describe what happens to the body slowly over time as the effects of posture and lifestyle habits change the physical structure, and "dented" is a good description of what happens to the body as a result of traumatic incidents, from birth trauma to falls at the playground to car accidents and the like.

The Forgiving Nature of Youth

Because of the forgiving nature of youth, we often make the mistake of thinking that our bodies are much more resilient than they actually are. Most of us go through the first half of life living relatively free of pain, and so we start to take our bodies for granted. But our younger bodies haven't had as much time to get folded and dented and to accumulate strain as our older bodies have. Add to this the fact that we're generally more active when we're young, and have more supple, pliable bodies, and it makes sense that our youthful bodies are able to do a very good job of adapting to and compensating for the stresses and strains that modern life dishes out.

It's a testament to the human body that in the face of structural compromise and misalignment—either from the subtle changes in posture that occur as we age or from the sudden falls or accidents that happen—it makes some amazing and complex adjustments in order to function as best it can. To avoid chronic knee or hip pain, for instance, your body will subtly shift the way you move in an attempt to avoid the pain without your even being aware of it. Our compensatory mechanisms are likely tied to a survival instinct, as there was a time in history when if you couldn't keep up with the migrating tribe you may very well have been left behind to fend for yourself! Whatever the origin, the end result is the body's ability to continue to function in the face of change while remaining as pain-free as possible.

Over time, however, it becomes harder and harder for the body to keep up with the demands that misalignment and tension place upon it. Eventually, it breaks down and you wake up one morning with myriad aches, pains, and health challenges, and an inability to do many of the things you once enjoyed.

The "Check Engine" Light

Of course there were warning signs, but the truth is that most of us pay more attention to the care and maintenance of our cars than we do to the care and maintenance of our own bodies. We ignore our own "check engine" warnings. Every time you get an ache or a pain, a twinge in a knee or soreness in your neck, your body is signaling you to pay attention to it or suffer more serious consequences down the road. We brush these warnings off as insignificant, however, because they usually last only a day or two or they get better after taking a couple of over-the-counter pain relievers. But for how long would you ignore the "check engine" light on your car's dashboard?

Following along with the car analogy, anyone who's ever bought tires, especially for an older car that likely has some minor alignment issues, knows that if you don't properly maintain the tires they'll wear out faster and need replacement long before expected. Your body is no different in its need for proper maintenance in order to avoid premature wear and tear. Without preventive measures and regular maintenance, the human body continues to become misaligned, accumulate stresses and strains, and lose its ability to adapt to and compensate for the demands of our lives.

Health Is a Dynamic Process

The simple truth is that the state of your health, of which your musculoskeletal system is a key component, is not static. It's not the same today as it was yesterday or will be tomorrow. *You're either moving toward health or, by default, moving away from it.* That's why when a patient comes into my office with a new onset of neck or back pain and says in wonderment, "But I didn't do anything unusual or different," I reply, "And that's the problem!" What I mean, of course, is that the body is changing over time, becoming tighter and more misaligned, and will eventually break down even while doing the same old things if you're not taking care to prevent the breakdown from happening. It may be the thousandth revolution of the bike pedal that month, or the hundredth weed you hunch over and pull that week, or the tenth time you lift your grandchild that day that finally creates the tear, the inflammation, or the spasm. *Just because you've done something many times in the past without consequences doesn't mean you can get away with it forever.* Just because you currently have no obvious physical complaints doesn't mean that your body isn't suffering on some level.

I recall one of my patients once proclaiming in shocked disbelief, "He died of a heart attack and he wasn't even sick!" But just because someone looks fine and has no current complaints doesn't mean that he or she doesn't have underlying problems. It doesn't mean that he or she can expect to go on without symptoms or illness indefinitely. Whoever the unfortunate man was who died without obvious warning, he was certainly sick. A heart attack doesn't just happen out of the blue, and neither does a herniated disc, the need for a hip replacement, or the average case of shoulder pain.

Though we cannot see the day-to-day changes that are occurring, it's an illusion to think that they're not happening and that we're maintaining the status quo. I was reminded of this recently when I saw a friend of mine whom I hadn't seen in about 15 years. I remember being somewhat shocked at how old he looked; his hair was thinning, his boyish look was long gone. It wasn't until much later that I realized he probably had the same reaction upon seeing me. In my own eyes, of course, I hadn't changed at all. But although we don't see it in ourselves as readily, you can be sure that our bodies—inside and out—are changing.

The Real Problem: Friction & Tension

To the majority of people, the most obvious and disturbing problem of a body that has been gripped or molded over time is the pain that eventually occurs. Though some will ignore it for a while, pain is usually the motivator that gets people to finally realize that something is wrong and to seek help for their condition.

Though not as readily apparent, there are potentially more serious problems associated with the molding of the body beyond the pain and limitation of activity that people experience. After all, the pain and everything that follows is really just a symptom of an underlying problem. The real problem is the friction and tension that are causing the disabilities.

Many middle-aged and older patients initially experience friction as a new sound their body makes when they move: grinding, clicking, or popping noises from their neck when they turn their head, from their shoulder when they reach for something, or from their knees when they squat down. As it progresses, tension in the body becomes a new inability to move in ways that people previously took for granted. The inability to bend over easily to put on shoes, difficulty turning the head to look over the shoulder when backing up a car, and trouble reaching the arm behind when putting on a jacket are all frequent complaints.

What many patients may not realize is that the friction in the body that they initially experience as a new sound together with the tension that limits movement can slowly wear and quickly tear the joints and soft tissues of the body, setting the stage for an inevitable breakdown. As a result of those rounding shoulders, for example, tension is created in the muscles that make up the shoulder joint—tension that eventually becomes tendinitis or a rotator cuff tear. A consequence of walking with one or both feet turned out, another very common habit, is abnormal friction in the hip and knee joints, resulting in the degeneration of cartilage and the meniscal tears that I see in my office in alarming numbers and at an increasingly early age. Stiffness in the lumbar spine from too much sitting forces the pressure from lifting a suitcase to herniate, or "blow out," the discs between the vertebrae.

The Effect on Your Organs

As if the breakdown of the musculoskeletal system weren't bad enough, there's another potential problem with friction and tension that's even more serious. Simply put, if left unchecked, the molding of the human frame can negatively affect the healthy functioning of the vital contents that live within it. The health and vitality of your blood vessels, nerves, and organs, for instance, depend heavily on the condition of the body that houses them. It can be no other way.

Advanced scoliosis, for example, a condition that by altering the spine changes the shape of the rib cage, directly affects the functioning of the organs that reside within the rib cage. Logical, right? Remember the envelope stuffed into your mailbox with the bent and damaged contents? All organs live within the framework of the body and rely on its shape (and protection!) to function properly. If a blood vessel, nerve, or organ is forced to change its position or otherwise accommodate itself to a misaligned and tight body, disastrous consequences—though slow to appear—can occur. In the case of severe scoliosis, the change in the shape of the spine and rib cage inevitably harms health (since structure and function go hand in hand), whether it's through compression of a lung or interference with the healthy functioning of the heart. It may even shorten the life expectancy of the individual.

Unfortunately, the potentially harmful effects of an impaired frame on internal organs aren't limited to cases of advanced scoliosis. We think of our bodies as tough and rugged, but they're really more like Swiss watches—they're finely tuned instruments with many delicate working parts inside. Move a bone or ligament a millimeter to the left—the result of rounded shoulders and a slumping back, say—and it can pinch a nerve or a nutrient-carrying artery, sowing the seeds of disease.

YOUR ARTERIES ARE LIKE GARDEN HOSES

Suppose you had a large garden with an underground irrigation system. Now let's say that through some mechanism—a burrowing animal, for example—a rock under the garden was moved an inch to the left and came to rest against one of the irrigation hoses, not fully compressing it but impeding it enough to decrease the flow of water by 50%. The section of the garden that receives its nourishment from that particular hose might do well enough for a while, but at some point it will become apparent that the plants in that section aren't doing as well as in the rest of the garden. Maybe their blossoms become sparse or their foliage gets a yellowish cast. Maybe stems and branches become lanky or brittle. Basically, it becomes clear that this area of the garden is slowly dying.

This is the kind of process that is likely happening in the human body all the time, and it's one of the causes of chronic aches, pains, and disease. Perhaps one of your bones or muscles has been displaced a millimeter to one side—through a fall you took on the ice or as a result of postural changes over time—and it's come to rest against one of your blood vessels. Over time, the area that the blood in this vessel is designed to nourish, whether a muscle, an organ, or a brain cell, will begin to slowly wither. Eventually, this will result in a serious problem. As with the garden, it can be so subtle that you don't even notice it for quite a long time—until one day it becomes so obvious that you can't avoid it.

The Old-Age Center

The upper back region has been referred to as the "old-age center" by osteopathic physicians for many years. The nickname comes from the observation that older patients, who have a generally high level of misalignment, stiffness, and tension in their upper backs, frequently also start to experience problems with their hearts and lungs. We've already discussed two of the possible explanations for this association: the fact that a change in the rib cage due to poor posture or scoliosis can negatively affect the organs housed within them; and the likelihood that the pinching of nutrient-carrying arteries that course throughout the region contributes to a "withering garden" effect.

There's a third, though debated, possible explanation for a misaligned and tight upper back creating problems for the heart and lungs. You're probably familiar with what happens when a *peripheral nerve* (one that leads to an extremity) gets pinched. You may have even experienced the resulting numbness, tingling, or radiating pain yourself. Carpal tunnel syndrome and sciatica are examples of painful conditions that can occur when peripheral nerves get pinched.

What you may not know, however, is that *autonomic nerves* can also get pinched. Unlike peripheral nerves, autonomic nerves exit the spine and travel to things called ganglia or plexuses, which are intermediary or relay centers for nerves. The relay centers send information to organs (rather than limbs) and are vital to their proper functioning. The autonomic nerves that exit the spine in the upper back travel to the intermediary centers for the heart and lungs and are responsible for, among other things, the heart's rate of contraction and the size of the airways of the lungs. Interference with the function of those upper back nerves, therefore, could ultimately create disturbances for the heart and lungs.

A Vicious Cycle

A gripped and molded body consumes a lot of its available energy in the process of adapting, compensating, and attempting to heal itself. As a consequence, there's less on hand to just get you through the day. Additionally, the tension inherent in a gripped body can directly or indirectly result in a depressed mood, impaired concentration and memory, poor quality of sleep, and a lack of motivation to act in healthy ways. When you're not feeling 100%, the desire to exercise, stretch, or eat well can be lacking. Unfortunately, this creates a vicious cycle in which pain and problems continue to worsen and recovery time is prolonged. It isn't until their pain decreases that most people come to realize how many other areas of their lives had been negatively affected by their deteriorating condition. Happily, as things begin to get better, many people frequently discover that they have a lot more energy than they used to.

Whether the molding of the human frame results in the degeneration of structures like tendons and joints; in compressing and restricting nerves and nutrient-carrying blood vessels; or in altering the environment where vital organs live, it ultimately leads to premature wear and tear, pain and dysfunction, and more than likely the inability of the body's organs to function correctly—all of which in turn eventually lead to chronic disease. A depressed mood, poor sleep, and lack of energy add insult to the injury.

And wait, there's another crucial reason to break the grip on the body and address issues of mis-alignment and friction: Many well-intentioned middle-aged and older people who begin an exercise routine for cardiovascular health soon find that their knees, hips, or other joints become painful, sending them to the sidelines. *Repetitive movements performed with a misaligned and tight body are a recipe for trouble*, especially if the exercise is high-impact. If you haven't been exercising regularly and begin an exercise routine in your 40s or beyond, it's imperative to keep your body stretched, loose, and better aligned. Otherwise, in spite of all your good intentions, you're just asking for trouble.

BRUSHING AND FLOSSING FOR YOUR BODY

We all understand how the accumulation of plaque and tartar leads to tooth and gum disease. And we all understand that in order to prevent disease and maintain the health of your mouth, it's important to get periodic care and cleanings from your dentist and dental hygienist. Understanding alone, of course, isn't nearly enough. You must take daily action as well, brushing and flossing your teeth to keep your mouth healthy.

It's no different with your body. A daily care and maintenance routine is just as important to keep your body from accumulating its own form of plaque. Fortunately, "brushing and flossing" for your body doesn't need to be any more complicated or time-consuming than brushing and flossing your teeth, and it can cure and prevent your body's aches and pains, keep you happier and healthier, and result in longevity and an improved quality of life. What a bargain!

End Everyday Pain

The movement program I prescribe takes ten minutes a day or less to complete and can fit into any-body's lifestyle. And while there certainly are degenerative conditions that cannot be reversed, I've often been amazed at the body's ability to heal. I once taught a patient with chronic neck pain and arthritis a few simple stretches and had her buy a new pillow that was the proper size. I encouraged her to change some of her postural habits, which she did, and her neck pain, which she had lived with for several years, went away in a few days! Although most cases won't resolve that quickly, it often takes only a minor adjustment, or a 5% to 10% change in a tight body, for relief to begin.

CHAPTER TWO

The Hammer:
Targeted Movement

*The doctor of the future will give no medication, but will
interest his patients in the care of the human frame...*

—Thomas A. Edison

Now that you have an understanding of how life in the modern world grips and molds the human frame over time, creating the misalignment and tension that result in wear and tear, chronic pain, and other medical problems, it's time to turn our attention to prevention and cure. While we'll talk more about the importance of habit modifications and visits to an outside practitioner in later chapters, it's time to turn our attention to the targeted movements.

Taken together, targeted stretching, strengthening, and range-of-motion exercises form such a powerful breaking-the-grip tool that I've dubbed them "The Hammer." Nothing else you can do will have a more potent effect in undoing the unhealthy molding of our frames that our work and play habits create. Stretching releases the tension in the body that sustains the grip, targeted strengthening helps return the body to an improved alignment, and range-of-motion exercises loosen and lubricate the soft tissues and joints. All of this translates into a body that's looser and, as I like to say, has more "space" in it. A body with more space in it has the ability and freedom to maneuver itself, to accommodate to the physical challenges of life without causing pain and injury, and to self-correct, which is its very nature.

When you lift a child, for example, the forces from lifting are delivered to your lumbar spine, discs, and lower back muscles, among other places. If your lower back is misaligned and tight as a result of too much sitting, for example, then those forces cannot be evenly spread out and absorbed by the body as designed. Instead, they'll be focused at one particularly tight and vulnerable spot, eventually resulting in a herniated disc, torn ligament, muscle spasm, or other unhappy outcome. Said another way, a tight and restricted body has no wiggle room, no ability to accommodate not only to the demands of such things as lifting, but also to the simple activities of daily life.

A word of caution: Because stretching, strengthening, and range-of-motion exercises have such a powerful impact on the body, people who have suffered recent physical trauma—especially trauma involving fractures of the bone, tears of the soft tissues, or obvious inflammation—should avoid them until fully healed. It's also important for pregnant women, people with osteoporosis, cancer, or other serious medical illness to check with their healthcare provider before embarking on any sort of exercise routine.

Stretching

It isn't unusual for new patients to tell me that they don't stretch because they tried it in the past and it didn't work; it didn't fix their problem or make their pain go away. If that's been your experience, or you've been discouraged from trying because you've heard that from someone you know, you need to realize a couple of things.

First, by far the most common reason that people don't get results is because either they don't do the right stretches, or they don't stretch correctly, or both. In all my years of treating patients, I can honestly say that I've only met a handful of people who did the necessary stretches—and keep in mind I only recommend a few for each area—and held them for the correct amount of time. There's a lot of incomplete and incorrect information out there.

In addition, for a small subset of people, no amount or type of stretching will be effective until they get some hands-on help from an outside practitioner. If the muscles, or the bones that they attach to, are extremely tight or misaligned, stretching will meet too much resistance from the body to be of much help. This is another example of why it often takes a couple of tools to treat the body successfully.

For effective stretching, I recommend *static stretches* because they're easy to do, familiar to most everyone, and have been proven to be effective. An example of a static stretch is one where you bend at the waist and reach for your toes, holding the position steady for a certain number of seconds. In a static stretch you remain still. Forget the bouncing and the pulling. Here are some other important points:

1. **Hold the stretch** for approximately 30 seconds if you're younger than 65 and closer to 60 seconds if you're 65 or older. Holding a stretch for a shorter period of time has been shown to be less effective.

2. **Do each stretch one time**, once a day, every day of the week. Though you may have to hold a stretch longer than you're used to, the good news is that doing several repetitions of each stretch, which a lot of people recommend, doesn't appear to improve the outcome significantly. "One and done," as they say.

3. **Stretch every day**. Although there are studies that show results with fewer days of stretching a week, doing them daily makes good sense. First, when you do something daily it becomes automatic; you don't have to decide whether or not you can skip that day. And second, remember that health is not static—you're either improving it or it's declining. We're adding to our mold every day!

The stretching, strengthening, and range-of-motion exercises that I prescribe *have been targeted* to the most commonly tight and molded areas of the body. They're easy to do and few in number. Few in number, however, does not mean ineffective! I've worked out the 80/20 rule (the common wisdom that holds that 80% of your results will come from 20% of what you do) as it applies to stretching, and I've boiled down your daily allotment of stretches to the 20% that I've seen produce the very best and fastest results. Over time, you can add more if you'd like.

Limited (for Now) Strengthening

Strengthening has an important role to play in the health of the human musculoskeletal system. Maintaining overall muscle tone and bone density as we age is crucial if we're to maintain our ability to function fully. For our purposes, however, I recommend that you start out strengthening just a few specific muscles that have typically weakened as a result of the molding process. Combined with the stretches and other tools, this targeted strengthening will help to break the grip on the body more quickly, correcting posture and improving health.

Temporarily limiting strengthening exercises to the few I suggest is important for several reasons. First, I want you to get results with the least amount of homework necessary, making it easier for you to get started and keep going. Second, utilizing the tools outlined in this book will improve your alignment and reduce tension in the body, which will *automatically* make you stronger. (I'll spare you the physics lecture, but suffice it to say that aligned muscles naturally perform better.) And, finally, engaging in random strengthening exercises with a tight and misaligned body can lead to increased asymmetry and more stress—and injury—on the already tight muscles, tendons, ligaments, and joints. More stress is not our goal!

Said another way, a more-aligned and looser body that's the product of all tools will have an easier time with additional strengthening exercises when and if they're added. My recommendation, therefore, is that you use the tools in this book for four to six weeks before adding other strengthening exercises.

Range-of-Motion Exercises

"Range of motion" (ROM) is a term used to describe the amount of available movement for each joint. Every joint in the body has a normal range that unfortunately tends to decrease as we age, especially if our tendency is to move less. Without preventive measures, the joints become stiff, pain and injury become more likely, and the ability to enjoy physical activity diminishes.

Unfortunately, studies demonstrate that we typically use only a small percentage of our available range of motion during daily activities like climbing stairs, bending to tie our shoes, or washing our hair.[1] The goal of dedicated range-of-motion exercises is to preserve, or increase if already reduced, the mobility of the joints by loosening the surrounding tendons and ligaments, and by stimulating joint lubrication. Done regularly, range-of-motion exercises can keep you moving effortlessly and painlessly.

PAY YOURSELF FIRST

There's a fundamental concept in finance that says, "Pay Yourself First." What this means is that you should put a little money from every paycheck into your savings account before spending it on other things, including your bills. The reason, of course, is so that over time you'll build wealth—or at least a nest egg—that will take care of you when you're older.

Pay Yourself First applies when it comes to your health, too. I use it to mean that you should spend a little time every day doing the things that over time will have the biggest impact on your health before you do the other things on your daily to-do list, however important they may be. Make stretching, strengthening, range-of-motion exercises, habit modifications (see page 87), and visits to outside practitioners (see page 98) a priority and they'll pay big dividends when you're older.

Eight Key Points

Keep the following eight points in mind as you engage in stretching, strengthening, and range-of-motion exercises:

1. Any time you start a new exercise routine you should proceed slowly until your body becomes accustomed to it. By slowly, I mean engaging your body with less intensity (like using less weight or doing fewer repetitions). I don't mean being inconsistent and sporadic.

2. Consistency is important when starting a new routine so that your body gets accustomed to the changes you're creating. Stopping and starting makes it harder for your body to break the old mold and move into a better, lasting arrangement.

3. When stretching, strengthening, and doing range-of-motion exercises, it's fine to feel a little discomfort, a warming, or even a mild tingling sensation as the muscles and joints become engaged. Exercising, however, should never create significant pain or numbness. If lasting pain, numbness, or soreness occurs, either as you're doing the exercise or later on, stop and rest the area for a couple of days and then begin again more slowly.

4. When performing a certain number of repetitions of a strengthening exercise—let's say 15—you must use enough weight or resistance so that doing a 16th repetition would be very difficult while maintaining good form. In other words, if you can do 15 repetitions quite easily, the muscle isn't challenged enough to get stronger.

5. Be careful but not fearful. Many patients have told me that they're afraid to do any form of exercise because their friends or their family members keep warning them about injury. But the body needs flexibility and movement! Just start slowly and consult an outside practitioner if you'd like guidance.

6. If you're prone to dizziness or have balance problems, always do your exercises on the floor, in a chair, or with someone by your side assisting you.

7. The best time to stretch is *now!* If you can exercise at the same time each day, it may help you to remember, but otherwise, do it whenever it's convenient for you. In the morning, late at night, or anytime in between, it doesn't matter. As long as they're done correctly, stretching and range-of-motion exercises can be a good way to warm up the body, to cool it down, or to give yourself a break from other activity (or non-activity).

8. Avoid the common pitfall of waiting to do your exercises until you're in pain or otherwise having problems. A regular routine done even when you're feeling well will prevent the old problems from returning and new ones from starting. *Stretch every day!*

Once you get started, stretching, strengthening, and range-of-motion exercises will most likely become a habit that you'll enjoy. Because you'll feel better, you'll never want to go back to your old, tight ways. Habits do take time to form, however (popular wisdom says it takes 21 days to lock in a new habit), so while you should try to be consistent, don't be discouraged if in the beginning you don't always remember to stretch. Stick with it and it will eventually become a pleasurable habit.

CHAPTER THREE
Zone 1: The Upper Body
Head, Neck, Shoulders, & Upper Back

Physical structure is the basis of medicine.

—Hippocrates

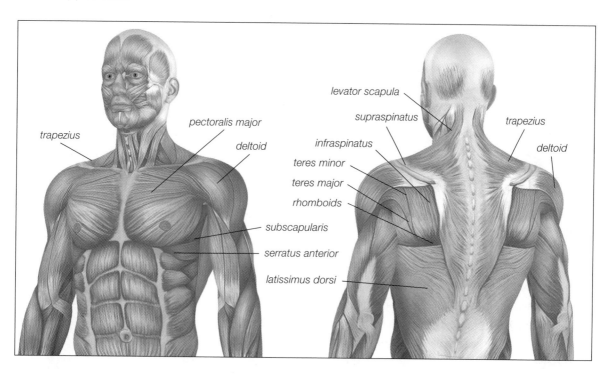

Aches, pains, and problems of the upper body are everyday occurrences for millions of people in the United States. Problems from the upper body interfere with a person's work and play and, all told, upward of *1 million people* every year elect to have surgery on their shoulders and necks.

As an osteopathic medical physician, I do believe it's important to seek an "official" diagnosis for your pain and other symptoms. But beyond that, as someone who specializes in the care of the human frame, I also know that modern medicine has almost no role to play in the average case of upper-body pain. Unless you have one of the rare and more serious conditions sometimes associated with headaches or neck pain, something your doctor would be alerted to by a radiologic study, all a modern medical doctor can do is offer you a prescription for anti-inflammatories and painkillers or perform invasive procedures. Neither of these options is likely to address the root cause of your pain, and both have potentially harmful side effects. So what's the real issue? Why do millions of people suffer chronic pain and get so little relief from the medical community? Read on and let's find out.

The Molding of the Upper Body—Wrapped Around an Imaginary Cylinder

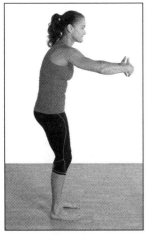

Figure 3-1

Zone 1 is a region that's greatly affected by the habits of modern living, and it always responds as a unit. Far too many of our activities—driving, reading, texting, working at the computer, cooking, and even sleeping in certain positions, to name a few—force us to wrap our upper bodies around what I often describe as an imaginary cylinder (figure 3-1).

The end results of maintaining this forward-reaching position throughout much of the day include a head that slowly moves forward, bringing the neck with it; shoulders that round, causing the shoulder blades to move away from the spine; and an upper back that becomes more prominent and, in extreme cases, forms a hump (figure 3-2). Perhaps more important to you in the short term, the forward molding also results in headaches, neck pain, and shoulder and upper-back pain.

Without anything to push on our arms and force our shoulders back (like the earth automatically does for four-legged animals), our upper bodies slowly, imperceptibly, but inevitably become "molded" in a forward direction. I observe this process all day long in my office as I treat people of various ages. In general, the older the patient, the more advanced the mold. In fact, with very few exceptions, I can close my eyes and place my hands underneath a new patient's upper back and tell his or her approximate age just from the resistance of the ribs and spine as I attempt to move them with my fingers. Almost without

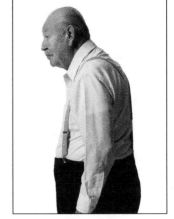

Figure 3-2

exception, the older the patient, the tighter and stiffer the upper back, and the more common the complaints of Zone 1–related pain.

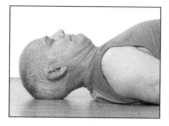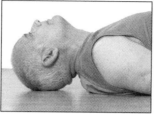

Figure 3-3. An individual lying face up—a normally aligned head (left) and one that has moved forward (right).

I first became aware of this upper-body molding process when my older patients, lying face up on my treatment table using the regular pillow I supplied, ended up with their heads tilting back, facing more toward my rear wall than straight up toward the ceiling as my younger patients did (figure 3-3). Typically, my older patients would then either bunch up the pillow I provided to make it fatter, or ask me for a second one. I soon realized that elevating the head made them more comfortable because it compensated for the fact that their whole upper body, as a unit, had moved more forward over time. When the weight of the head pulled it back down as they were lying on my table (while the shoulders remained forward, sometimes so much so that they weren't actually touching the table), they became extremely uncomfortable. In fact, the shoulders of some of these older patients had become so molded forward that it was literally impossible to move them back and down toward the more normally aligned position of my younger patients.

SELF-TEST: HOW FAR HAS YOUR HEAD MOVED FORWARD?

To get an idea of how far your head has moved forward, lie flat on the floor on your back, with the back of your head resting on the floor. If your chin is sticking up in the air and you're looking more behind you than straight up at the ceiling, your head has moved forward on your trunk.

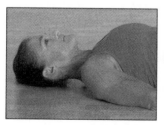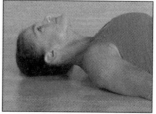

To get an idea of how rounded your shoulders are, look at yourself in a full-length mirror, with a relaxed posture, and count the number of knuckles you can see on the backs of your hands. If you can see more than two—the knuckles of the thumb and index finger—your shoulders are rounding forward, causing your arms and hands to turn inward.

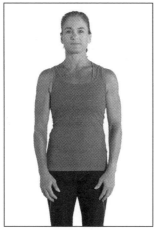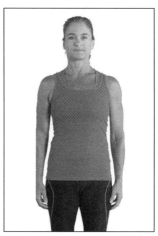

Left: Round shoulders, more knuckles visible. Right: Good posture.

Tense, Tight, & Strained

A forward-moving head and rounded shoulders are two outcomes of the molding process, a process that alters the position of the bones, muscles, tendons, and ligaments of the upper body from their original design, and in the process tightens and stresses them. Body workers call this misalignment, and the tension it creates becomes obvious to practitioners like me when we place our hands on the upper bodies of our patients.

Whether a patient appears in my office with headaches, neck pain, shoulder pain, upper-back pain, or not infrequently a combination of them, my experience is that it's as a result of this upper-body molding process. That includes those cases where a specific event—like raking leaves, carrying a suitcase, or lifting a child—triggered the pain, because in all likelihood the area was already vulnerable due to misalignment and tension.

I often compare a tight body to a bucket full to the brim with water, where any added stress becomes the drop that finally causes the bucket to overflow. Releasing tension from the body is like removing some of the water from the bucket, which as a result can now accept more without spilling over. My patients often discover to their surprise that their old reliable pain triggers don't have the same negative impact on the upper body that they used to once they've begun using the treatment tools that I recommend.

Common Complaints from Zone 1

While we're going to treat the whole upper body rather than break it into parts, let's first get a better understanding of the most-common localized complaints in this zone.

Headaches

Though they may seem somewhat removed, headaches are often rooted in problems of the musculoskeletal system. Regardless of their official medical classification (tension and migraine being the two most common), the vast majority of the headaches that my middle-aged and older patients suffer from are caused or exacerbated by misalignment and tension in the bones, muscles, and soft tissues of the upper body.

The classic presentation of a *tension headache*, the most common type of headache experienced by adults, is often described as pain that's dull and achy in nature, frequently arising from the neck or back of the head and wrapping around the head like a tight headband. Pain can begin early in the day and generally gets worse as the day progresses. Most physicians can understand and properly diagnose this type of headache as resulting from muscle tension.

The classic presentation of a *migraine headache*, the second most-common type of headache, is debilitating pain that's sharp or throbbing in nature and affects the whole head or just one side of it. Migraines are often accompanied by side effects such as nausea and light sensitivity. Unlike with tension headaches, many modern physicians fail to see the relationship of the musculoskeletal system to migraine headaches. But while the cause of migraines remains largely unknown, it bears repeating that the muscles, soft tissues, and bones of the upper body are intimately connected with the structures within the head and influence, among other things, the functioning of the blood vessels, nerves, and other pain-sensitive tissues thought to be involved.

While most of the focus in migraine treatment is on those things that trigger them, attention should also be placed on the underlying conditions that may predispose individuals to get them in the first place. Paying attention to the underlying conditions, in fact, is a way of focusing on the cure. Like other practitioners who treat the musculoskeletal system, I've successfully treated all headache types, migraines included, by directly releasing tension in the upper body and by teaching my patients how to do it on their own.

Although some medical textbooks and websites list a musculoskeletal cause for headaches (poor posture, for example), they typically don't address treatment in any depth because most physicians no longer have the skill to do hands-on work. The fact is, however, hands-on work has been proven to be successful in the treatment of headaches beyond a shadow of a doubt, as the following studies make clear:

> *Researchers at Northwestern Health Sciences University reviewed and analyzed scientific data from 22 studies involving 2,628 patients and concluded that spinal manipulation was effective at preventing both migraine headaches and headaches arising from the neck ("cervicogenic").[2] Neck exercises were also found effective for both short-term relief and long-term prevention of headaches arising from the neck.*

In a separate study, also performed at Northwestern Health Sciences University:

> *Researchers reviewed the results of nine randomized clinical trials involving 683 patients with chronic headaches and concluded that spinal manipulative therapy had an effect comparable to first-line prophylactic prescription medication for migraine and tension-type headaches.[3]*

Neck Pain

Neck pain is most commonly described as mild, irritating, achy, or stiff; occasionally it can be sharp and severe. It often results in a reduced range of motion, an example of which would be difficulty looking over the shoulder to back up the car. Most people cannot attribute the onset of neck pain to a specific event or incident, which makes sense because it's usually the insidious end result of poor alignment and tension.

A less-common type of neck pain is commonly termed "whiplash" and occurs in situations where the neck has been traumatized. Most commonly associated with car accidents, whiplash can also occur in many other types of accidents, including slips and falls. Regardless of whether the accident occurred yesterday or 30 years ago, unless the spine and soft tissues of the neck and upper body have been properly treated, accident trauma can cause recurring pain.

It's not unusual for neck-pain patients to blame their condition on arthritis, a disc problem, or a pinched nerve. One thing is certain: There's a lot of misinformation out there about the sources of pain. In my experience, arthritis, disc problems, and other such conditions are rarely the cause of my patients' pain, either the dull and chronic variety or the acute and debilitating type. In fact, many people with no neck pain at all walk around with these common diagnoses, as evidenced by the following study:

The Orthopedic Department of Surgery at the George Washington University Medical Center studied the cervical MRIs of 63 healthy volunteers who had *no history of neck pain or disability* and found:

- Overall cervical spine abnormalities were reported in 28% of the volunteers over 40 years old.

- Herniated discs were seen in 10% of those under 40 and 5% of those over 40 years old.

- Stenosis was seen in 20% of those over 40 years old.

- Evidence of disc degeneration or narrowing in almost 60% of those over 40 and 25% in those younger than 40 years old.

- Compression of the spinal cord and bone spurs were also seen on the MRIs.[4]

Radiological findings such as arthritis, bulging or herniated discs, stenosis, and bone spurs are easy to target as pain-producing culprits because they appear on the neck X-rays and MRIs of so many older people—including those without any complaints of pain! The significance of these findings, therefore, may be that to some extent they reflect the level of misalignment and tension building in the body. In other words, *they are the end results of the problem and not the cause of them*.

Practitioners who use their hands to diagnose and treat their patients follow the old adage "treat the patient and not the lab result," which in this example might mean treat the muscle tension and the stiff spine and don't worry about the often-misleading X-ray or MRI report. In the process, patients often get better even if their X-ray and MRI results stay the same. (The imaging results may also improve, of course; a more supple spine has an easier time reabsorbing a disc bulge, for example.) As proof of the hands-on approach, we can look at the following study:

> *The Sunnybrook Health Sciences Centre in Canada reviewed 31 randomized controlled trials to examine the effectiveness of conservative treatment for mechanical neck disorders. After analyzing the data, the authors concluded that there was strong evidence of benefit utilizing a "multimodal" approach, combining exercise (stretching and strengthening) with mobilization or manipulation for subacute and chronic mechanical neck disorders, with or without headaches, in the short and long term.[5]*

Shoulder Pain

Shoulder pain is typically described as dull and achy. It's usually located around the top of the shoulder, and in advanced cases can radiate down the arm into the biceps or as far as the forearm. Dull and achy pain can quickly become sharp pain when the arm is moved into certain positions, such as raising it overhead to reach for something, or placing it behind the back as when trying to put on a shirt or a jacket. Pain in bed while trying to sleep frequently occurs as the problem progresses.

Some adult patients who are plagued by shoulder pain arrive at my office with no previous work-up, while others, after having seen their family doctor or an orthopedic specialist, come with a specific diagnosis such as:

Tendinitis/Tendinopathy: inflammation or strain of a shoulder muscle tendon

Bursitis: inflammation of the fluid-filled sacs (bursa) that surround the shoulder and cushion its movement

Impingement syndrome: pinching of the shoulder tendon(s) or bursa in the subacromial space (the space under the "knob" on the top of the shoulder)

Rotator cuff tear: a tear of one or more of the four main tendons of the shoulder

Regardless of the diagnosis, the soft tissues of these patients' shoulders are irritated and, barring rare physical shoulder trauma, got that way at least in part due to the rounding process. Unless that fact is addressed, the problem will be slow to resolve and will likely return no matter what interventions are taken.

SLOWLY FRAYING ON THE ROCK'S EDGE

The image I often use to describe the muscle-straining process that results from shoulder rounding comes from the scene in the old Western movie where our hero is descending down a cliff using a rope, which to our dismay is seen to be slowly fraying as it rubs on the rock's edge. The suspense mounts as one after another of the rope's fibers rip. Eventually, the last fiber tears and the rope breaks completely—but not before our hero has managed to get close enough to the bottom to be able to land safely and continue on in the movie.

All of the many and varied activities that we engage in with our arms out in front of us pull the shoulders forward, pinching and straining the muscle fibers, while you, like the cowboy rappelling down the cliff, are unaware of the impending doom. As this has been a gradually developing process, the actual event that ends up causing the shoulder injury can be so minimal as to not even be remembered by the patient. Fortunately, with awareness of this process and a few preventative measures, you can land safely at the bottom of the cliff—with your shoulder muscles intact!

To understand how the rounding of the shoulder leads to pain and problems requires a brief anatomy lesson. There are four major muscles of the shoulder whose tendons collectively form a "cuff"—the rotator cuff—that's responsible for stabilizing the shoulder and allowing all of the amazingly complex movements of the arm. The vast majority of shoulder pain and problems, however, involves one particular rotator cuff tendon, the *supraspinatus* tendon, and occurs in an area of the shoulder called the subacromial space, the space below the acromion. When this subacromial space narrows, it pinches, or "impinges," the structures within it (figure 3-4). Not only does the supraspinatus tendon lie within the subacromial space, the subacromial bursa also sits in there, which explains why it's the bursa most frequently irritated.

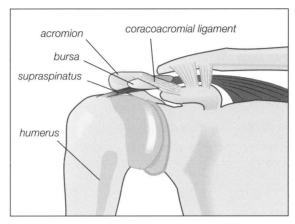

Figure 3-4

So what causes the subacromial space to narrow and cause all those shoulder problems? Well, studies have shown that when the shoulder blades move away from the spine (an outcome of forward rounding shoulders) or when the upper back rounds (creating a hump, which also coincides with the forward movement of the shoulders), the subacromial space gets smaller.[6, 7] It stands to reason, therefore, that treatment aimed at exercising the shoulder, releasing tension, and improving posture has an important role to play in relieving pain and improving function. Treatment aimed at the effects of impingement, on the other hand, through such modalities as surgery, would seem to be less effective. As evidenced below, studies bear this out:

A 2009 study conducted at the Vanderbilt Shoulder Center reviewed the results from 11 randomized controlled trials to evaluate the role of exercise in treating rotator cuff impingement. The authors concluded that the data demonstrated statistically and clinically significant effects of exercise on pain reduction and improved function for patients with rotator cuff impingements.[8]

In contrast, a 2008 study conducted by the Cochrane Musculoskeletal Group reviewed the medical research database to determine the effectiveness and safety of surgery for rotator cuff disease (including rotator cuff tears, impingement syndrome, and calcific tendinitis) versus non-surgical approaches. After analyzing the results of 14 randomized clinical trials involving 829 participants, the authors determined that "we cannot draw firm conclusions about the effectiveness or safety of surgery for rotator cuff disease."[9]

Upper Back Pain

Upper back pain can be nagging and dull in quality, but more often is described as sharp and stabbing—like a "knife in the back." The most common area of pain occurs slightly to one side of the spine in the area between the shoulder blades, right and left sides being equally represented. The pain is usually brought on by movements of the arm on the involved side or by turning the head, but it can be triggered by something as simple as taking a deep breath. While some patients can't trace the origin of their upper back pain to a specific activity, many others can describe the exact event that initiated the pain.

The most common cause of upper back pain is—I bet you know what I'm going to say here— rounding forward of the shoulders. As they round, the shoulder blades are pulled away from the spine of the upper back, creating tension, weakness, and strain on the muscles (the rhomboids) that connect the two (figure 3-5).

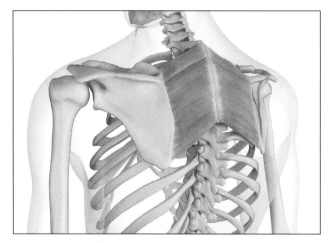

Figure 3-5. Rhomboid muscles

What's more disturbing than the resulting pain, however, are the negative consequences that upper back stiffness and tension can have on the healthy functioning of the vital organs that reside just on the other side of it, within the rib cage. It bears repeating that osteopathic doctors sometimes refer to the upper back area as "the old-age center" because they believe that many of the more serious problems of old age, including problems of the heart and lungs, are the result of chronic tension in the upper backs of their older patients. Remember how this impacts the arteries, the nerves, and the structure that houses these organs? Reducing this tension, therefore, may have far-reaching benefits beyond just pain relief!

Other Zone 1 Problems Related to Molding

The molding of the upper body and the resulting grip it places on its component parts may be responsible for other problems that many middle-aged and older people experience. They include:

1. Numbness and/or Tingling of the Hands

The nerves that travel to the hands begin in the neck and upper back and travel past the front of the shoulder on their way to the fingertips. Misalignment and tension anywhere along this course can put pressure on, or "pinch," these nerves, creating numbness and/or tingling in the fingers. Once serious but rare causes of numbness have been ruled out, hands-on treatment and stretching can be undertaken, and these frequently reduce or eliminate the symptoms.

2. Swallowing Difficulties

Some of my older patients have reported difficulty swallowing food or pills as they've gotten older. Though there are serious medical conditions that may lead to this problem, an often-overlooked cause is the misalignment of the head and neck. As the head moves forward on the trunk, the throat, which courses down the neck on its way into the trunk, has no choice but to alter its position as well. This change in position can compromise the normal physiologic process of swallowing—just like a kink in a garden hose inhibits water from flowing smoothly.

3. Jaw Pain

Jaw pain is frequently the result of misalignment and tension in the head and neck. The temporo-mandibular joints (TMJ) are located on both sides of the head near the ears, where the jaw bone (mandible) connects to the skull. Any asymmetry of the neck, head, or jaw, can result in TMJ dysfunction and pain. Many people first experience this asymmetry as a change in their bite, some-times necessitating dental work. Improving the posture of the upper body and reducing tension in the area often cures the problem.

4. Tremors

Tremors are involuntary shaking movements most commonly affecting one or both hands, or less frequently the head. Mild tremors are not uncommon experiences for older people, and although they can be symptoms of underlying disease or side effects of medication, medical work-ups are often negative, with no cause or explanation given for the onset of the condition. Of course, one explanation is that tension in the upper spine compresses and irritates the nerves, causing them to malfunction. Reducing the tension may improve this condition and mitigate its symptoms.

5. Vertigo

The most common form of vertigo, benign paroxysmal positional vertigo (BPPV), is an inner-ear disorder that's triggered by changes in the position of the head. As the only major risk factor to developing BPPV is age, it's possible that the sensitive inner ear may be disturbed by the forward movement and asymmetric positioning of the head and neck that become more common as we age. Improving the posture of the upper body and reducing tension in the area may lessen symptoms.

6. A Sudden "Electric Shock" in the Neck

The feeling of an electric shock zapping up or down the neck is a complaint occasionally reported to physicians and chiropractors. The sensation most often happens with a sudden movement of the head or neck, like a quick turn of the head or a sneeze. While this is a potentially serious problem and should be evaluated medically, it's more often the result of a nerve being pinched in a misaligned and tight neck. Hands-on work and stretching often eliminate the problem.

Let's Get Started

While we may not want or be able to change the activities we engage in on a daily basis (like driving or working at a computer), and we can't avoid the accidental traumas and mishaps that occur, we *can* dedicate a few minutes every day to maintaining our human frame and improving the quality of our lives. As you embark on this program, it's important that you understand that studies have not only demonstrated that exercises work, but also that *home-based* exercises are often as effective at reducing pain and improving function as those supervised by a physiotherapist.[10, 11] So while I encourage you to get the help of knowledgeable outside practitioners like physical therapists for support and guidance, you need to do the exercises at home, too. No exercise program will help you unless you follow it!

ZONE 1 PROGRAM: The Upper Body

STRETCHING		
EXERCISE	REP	DURATION
Shoulder & Chest, page 32	1	:30
Upper Back, Shoulder, & Neck, page 34	1	:30
Neck, page 35	1	:30
STRENGTHENING		
Rhomboids, page 37	1	:30
RANGE-OF-MOTION		
Shoulder Rolls, page 38	1	:30
Total time of daily workout		2:30

The key to both curing and preventing upper body pain and problems is to do some targeted exercises to unwrap the upper body from the imaginary cylinder in front of it. The stretching exercises will *loosen* the shortened and tight muscles that form in front (the chest, front of the shoulders, and anterior neck) and the strengthening exercises will *strengthen* the lengthened and weakened muscles that result in back (between the shoulder blades). The range-of-motion exercises *lubricate* and *release tension* in the vertebrae, ribs, and shoulder joints. Taken together, these exercises improve posture and ease the strain on the region, allowing blood flow to improve, inflammation to be reduced, waste products to be removed, nerves to be free to conduct impulses unimpeded, muscles and other soft tissues to return to their original length and tone, and bulging discs to become reabsorbed.

NOTE: Make sure you've read Chapter Two (page 14) for important general information about the use of these exercises.

Hold all stretches a minimum of 30 seconds and do each at least once.

Shoulder & Chest Stretch

This stretch puts the imaginary cylinder behind you and is therefore one of the most important exercises you can do to reverse the rounding forward of the head and shoulders.

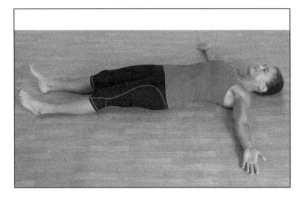

The Position: Lie on the floor face up and put your arms straight out to the sides.

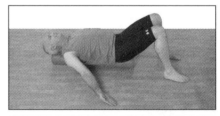

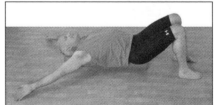

NOTE: If you don't feel a stretch in the shoulder or chest muscles when lying on the floor, try lying on a roll along the length of your spine. A rolled-up towel or foam bolster will do nicely. Your head should be supported by the roll itself or with a pillow of equal height. As long as you keep them on the floor, you can vary the position of your arms (lower toward your hips, higher toward your head) to stretch different parts of the chest and shoulder muscles.

ALTERNATE VERSION: Though not as effective (because your muscles are more relaxed when lying on the floor), this doorway version can be done when lying down is not convenient, like when at work.

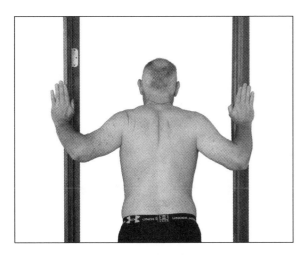

The Position: Stand with your feet shoulder-width apart on the inside of a doorway and gently lean forward, through the doorway, with arms out, elbows bent, and palms on the molding.

Try to feel your shoulder blades pinch together, coming closer to your upper back spine. Keep your head aligned with your trunk, not falling forward ahead of your body.

As with the floor version, you can vary the height of the arms on the sides of the door to stretch different parts of the chest and shoulder muscles.

Upper Back, Shoulder, & Neck Stretch

This is a great exercise to wake up a tired upper back. It helps to stretch the neck and spine and reverse the rounding forward of the shoulders.

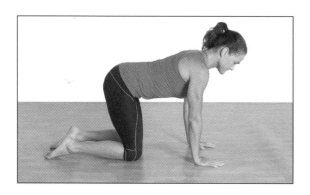

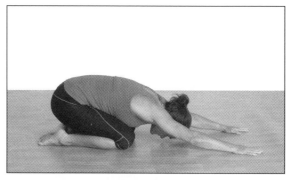

1. Start out by getting down on your hands and knees on all fours.

2. Now allow your hips and knees to bend further, bringing your butt lower toward the floor and extending your arms out in front of you. (In yoga this is known as child's pose.) You should feel the stretch in the upper arms, shoulders, and upper back.

STANDING VERSION: This version of the upper back and shoulder stretch is not quite as effective, but it's good for times when lying down is not convenient.

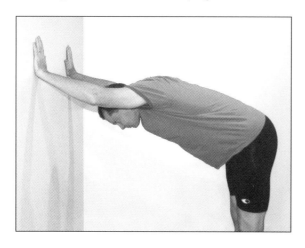

The Position: Stand with your feet shoulder-width apart, knees slightly flexed, and bend forward at the hips while keeping your lower back curve intact. Don't round your lower back. Maintain a solid base by keeping your hips above your knees, which are above your feet. Extend your arms straight out in front of you, parallel with the floor, and grab a wall, a dresser, a high counter—anything that's level with your outstretched arms. Your torso and legs will create an L shape. Now relax your head and upper body, allowing their weight to gently lower them between your arms toward the floor. You should feel the stretch in the upper arms, shoulders, and upper back.

Neck Stretch

This is an important stretch to help reverse the process of the head moving forward on the body. It also serves to elongate and properly situate the neck, creating more space between the vertebra for the discs, which counteracts the tendency for them to bulge or herniate.

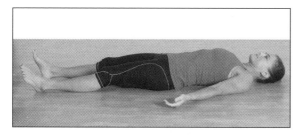

1. Lying flat on your back on the floor (or bed), let your head relax for a few seconds. *NOTE:* If your head has moved significantly forward on your body, this simple position may be too uncomfortable. If that's the case, place as thin a pillow as you're comfortable with under your head. You can also put a pillow under your knees if your lower back is uncomfortable in this position.

To perform the stretch, all you need to do is keep moving your fingers up, pushing—or sliding—the back of your head up, feeling the back of your neck elongating. You may also notice that this movement tilts your head down.

NOTE: The back of your head should remain in contact with the floor, or pillow, at all times—you're sliding the back of your head along the floor, not lifting it up off the ground.

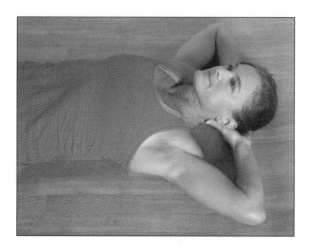

2. Now reach up and place the fingers of both hands in the space behind your neck, fingertips touching or fingers interlocked, and very gently move them up along the floor until they contact the back of your resting head.

SEATED OR STANDING VERSION: This version of the neck stretch is not quite as effective as the one done while lying down, since the muscles are not as relaxed when your head is erect, but it's good for times when lying down is not convenient.

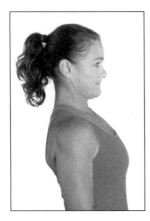 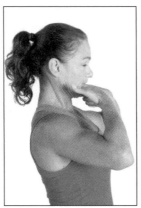

The Position: From a comfortable seated or standing position, look straight ahead and gently pull your head back, tucking your chin, and feeling the back of your neck lengthen. Though your chin will tilt down slightly, your goal is not to strictly nod your head down but to move it back, creating a double chin. You can use your hands to facilitate this action by gently pushing your chin back. You should feel the stretch at the back of the neck.

Hold or maintain all strengthening exercises a minimum of 30 seconds and do each at least once.

Rhomboids Exercise

The easiest, gentlest way to begin strengthening the upper body muscles is with isometric exercise. In this exercise, we target the rhomboid muscles, which become weaker as a result of the rounding of the shoulders. Strengthening them is essential to realigning the upper body and decreasing pain.

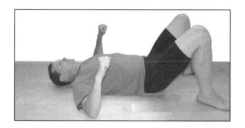

The Position: Lie on your back with your arms straight out to the side and your elbows bent 90 degrees. Your forearms should be perpendicular to the ground with your fists pointing up to the ceiling. Push your elbows into the floor, lifting your upper back slightly off the ground while squeezing your shoulder blades together toward the spine. Really feel your shoulder blades pinching together, doing the work of lifting you off the ground—rather than your arms and shoulders doing most of the work.

Hold for 3 seconds, then rest for a few seconds.

Repeat 10 to 12 times once a day, 3 times a week, with a day or two of rest in between sessions.

ALTERNATE VERSION: Though a little harder to feel the upper back muscles working, this version can be done when lying down isn't convenient, like when at work.

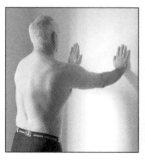 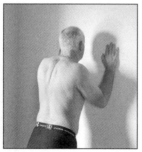

1. Begin with your hands against the wall, fingers pointing up, slightly below shoulder height, and your arms extended in front of you—keeping your shoulders back.

2. Pinch your shoulder blades together, moving them closer to your spine. Bend your elbows as you slowly move your body toward the wall. Keep your head and neck relaxed and straight.

When you reach the wall, slowly push off and back toward the starting position, keeping the shoulder blades pinched toward the middle the whole time. Each "wall push-up" should last about 10 seconds from beginning to end. Doing them slowly makes the muscles work harder, increasing their effectiveness.

Repeat 3 times once a day, 3 times a week, with a day or two of rest in between sessions.

Perform range-of-motion maneuvers a minimum of 30 seconds and do each at least once.

Shoulder Rolls

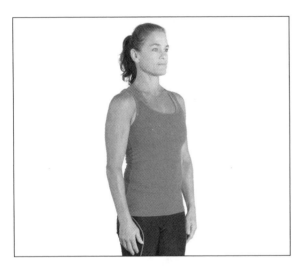 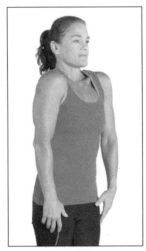 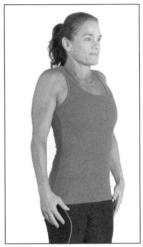

1. From a comfortable seated or standing position, relax your arms at your sides.

2. Slowly roll both of your shoulders forward and then backward 5 times in each direction. You should feel your upper back and ribs moving along with your shoulders.

Repeat several times throughout the day.

CHAPTER FOUR
Zone 2: The Lower Back

Treat the patient, not the X-ray.

—Anonymous

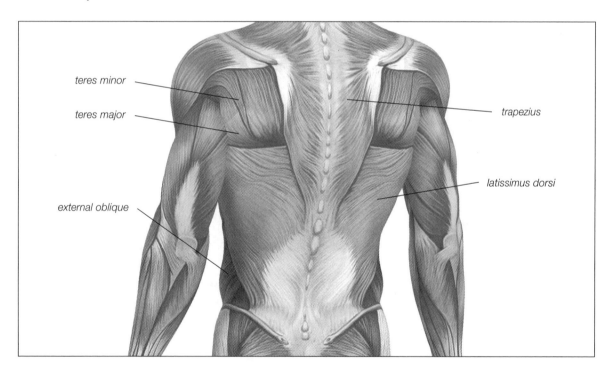

teres minor

teres major

trapezius

latissimus dorsi

external oblique

According to the National Institutes of Health's Low Back Pain Fact Sheet, nearly everyone at some point in his or her life will have lower back pain severe enough to interfere with their work or play. All told, the United States spends 50 billion dollars a year on this common ailment. What steps can you take to avoid—or stop—contributing to this massive sum? At the risk of sounding like a broken record, I'll repeat that while it's important to check in with your family physician for an "official" medical diagnosis, modern medicine has almost no role to play in the average case of lower back pain. Unless you have one of the rare and more serious conditions sometimes associated with lower back pain, something your doctor would be alerted to by any one of several red flags, all the modern medical doctor can do is offer you a prescription for anti-inflammatories, muscle relaxants, and painkillers, or perform invasive procedures, none of which address the real issue and all of which have potentially harmful side effects.

Description & Location

The most common area of lower back pain is a somewhat vague distribution on one side or across both sides of the lower back, slightly above the belt line (figure 4-1, point A). Less frequently, lower back pain can be located at a very well-defined spot, lower down below the belt line, to the right or left of the sacrum (figure 4-1, point B), which is the bone at the bottom of the spine. It's not unusual to experience other additional areas related to back pain including pain in the buttock or hip. Lower back pain itself is typically described as either sharp and debilitating with an accompanying feeling of fragility, or dull and annoying, like a toothache.

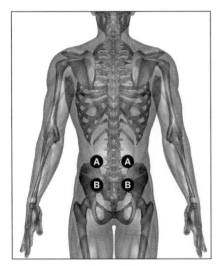

Figure 4-1

Lower back pain is often precipitated by a known specific event. Patients can usually describe exactly what they were doing—lifting a child, perhaps, or putting a suitcase in the car—when the pain began. In these cases the pain is often immediate and leaves the person feeling very vulnerable. Relief is often achieved by finding a position of comfort and staying immobile, like lying flat on your back on the floor with both knees bent. It can be close to impossible to straighten up, as from out of a chair, without pain.

At other times, patients cannot attribute their lower back pain to a specific event, as is the case when they go to bed without any known problem but wake up the next morning in pain. In these situations, the pain is typically dull and achy in character and progresses throughout the day.

The Molding of the Lower Back

Unlike what many people have been led to believe, lower back pain is rarely the result of arthritis, degenerative disease, bone spurs, spinal stenosis, disc bulges or herniations. (More on this in "Arthritis, Disc Disease, Spinal Stenosis, and Other Scapegoats" on page 49). The vast majority of lower back pain cases, regardless of the description of the pain or its location, are the result of misalignment and tension that in the lower back come about for two main reasons: 1) It's the meeting place of the upper and lower body and 2) we move too little and sit too much.

The Meeting Place: The lower back is a particularly vulnerable area of the human frame because it's the meeting place of the upper and lower halves of the body. It's influenced by those structures above it, like the head, shoulders, and rib cage, and by those below it, like the legs, hips, and pelvis.

As these areas themselves are typically misaligned, you could say it's the place where "twists" from above meet "twists" from below, just as the forces of a wringing washcloth meet in the middle.

If you look closely at yourself in the mirror from the front, back, and sides, you'll likely see some of these asymmetries yourself; few of us are spared them. As a lab exercise in osteopathic medical school, we dressed in shorts or

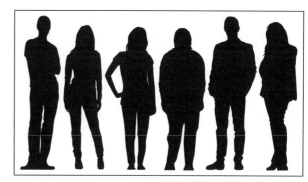

Figure 4-2. Common body misalignments

bathing suits and examined each other's bodies. The average age of the students in the class was 23 years old and yet we still saw countless examples of shoulders and pelvises that were not level, upper backs and shoulders that were rounding, feet and legs and that were turned out or rotated, and the like (figure 4-2). Unfortunately, these asymmetries and misalignments only become more advanced as people age, further influencing the lower back and resulting in acute and chronic lower back pain and problems.

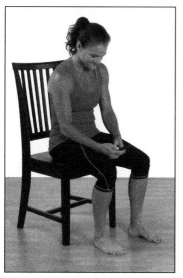

Figure 4-3

A Sedentary Lifestyle: The lower back is also vulnerable to pain and problems because life in the modern world tends to limit how much we're required to move while affording ample opportunity for sitting. Whether we're working at a desk, catching up with friends on Facebook, watching television, or driving in our cars, the result is the same: We're sitting way too much. In fact, it's almost as if our bodies are wrapped around an imaginary ball in front of our waist for most of the day and night (figure 4-3). The end result is the gradual molding and stiffening of the lower back and the pain and dysfunction that follow.

Take those 23-year-old medical students with their body asymmetries, add 30 years of being wrapped around an imaginary ball, and season with a general lack of awareness and attention to the process of molding, and voila! You've got legions of over-50-year-olds with tense, tight, and strained lower backs and 50 billion dollars a year spent on its treatment!

Lower back tension can affect both the lumbar spine and the muscles. Two groups of muscles (the hip flexors and the back extensors) are particularly vulnerable due to the imbalances that wrapping around the imaginary ball creates. Let's talk about them now and return to the lumbar spine later.

The Hip Flexor Muscles

The psoas muscles (pronounced *so-az*) begin at the lumbar spine, join forces with the iliacus muscles (pronounced *il-ee-ak-us*) inside the pelvis, and become the most powerful hip flexors of the body (figure 4-4).

Hip flexors are named as such because their main job is to flex your thigh up toward your trunk at the hip joint or, alternatively, raise your trunk up toward your thighs (going from a lying position to a sitting one). Unfortunately, we spend so much time in this flexed-hip position (wrapped around the imaginary ball) that these muscles get shorter, tighter, and weaker over time and are a frequent cause of acute and chronic lower back pain.

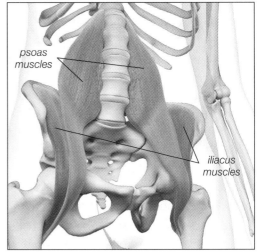

psoas muscles

iliacus muscles

Figure 4-4

OUR MOST POWERFUL AND VULNERABLE MUSCLE

The psoas muscles of the lower back, which run down both sides of the lumbar spine and through the pelvis on their way to the thighs, are two of the most powerful, important, and vulnerable muscles in the human body. You may be more familiar with the psoas muscles of the cow or pig, as they're a very popular cut of meat called the "tenderloin." The tenderloin's popularity stems from the fact that for meat eaters it's regarded as the tenderest cut of meat. Its tenderness can be explained by the fact that in four-legged animals the hind legs are almost always at a 90-degree angle to the spine, placing the psoas muscles in a shortened position that essentially does no work. Because it does little or no work, the muscle becomes soft, or tender.

In humans, by contrast, our two-legged upright arrangement requires the psoas muscles to be very active as they're responsible for helping us sit up, raise our legs, walk, bend, lift, carry, and kick. In the modern world, however, we spend so much time sitting—creating a similar angle between the spine and legs as in the four-legged animals—that our psoas muscles become shorter and weaker over time. When we finally ask the psoas muscles to do some work, like lift a child, move furniture, or play tennis on the weekend, they're often not up to the task and go into painful spasm, pulling the trunk sideways or forward, and in some cases making it difficult to even stand upright.

Unless we take steps to counteract the shortening of the psoas muscles from years spent sitting, not only are we apt to develop lower back pain and problems, we may also come to discover one day that we can't even stand fully erect anymore. When these valuable and vulnerable muscles can no longer achieve their normal length, neither can we! Fortunately, it only takes one easy stretch to help prevent this problem and you'll find it in the movement routines at the end of the chapter.

The Back Extensor Muscles

The deepest of the spinal erectors, the multifidus (pronounced *mul-tif-ih-dus*) muscle lies right up against the spine and is made up of smaller bundles of muscles that span one to several vertebrae each. It runs up the length of the spine, from the sacrum to the neck (figure 4-5).

The multifidus muscle does many jobs, two of the most important of which are stabilizing the spine and bending it backward. It, too, suffers when we wrap ourselves around that imaginary ball, becoming elongated and weak due to the position the spine typically assumes when sitting. Studies have not only demonstrated this weakness, but have also shown that strengthening the multifidus muscle can alleviate chronic lower back pain.

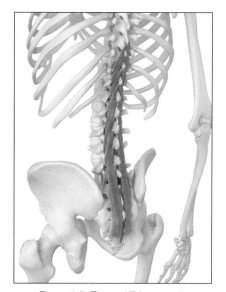

Figure 4-5. The multifidus muscle

> As reported in the journal Spine, researchers in the Netherlands set out to investigate whether or not isolated lumbar-extensor strengthening affected patients' self-reported chronic lower back pain status. The study concluded that just ten weeks of once-a-week strengthening "leads to clinically relevant improvements in functional status of men with chronic non-specific lower back pain."[12]

Two tools can help restore the multifidus muscle to a healthier state. The first is the strengthening exercise you'll find at the end of this chapter. The second is maintaining the correct position of the lumbar spine—also known as having good posture—discussed in Chapter Six.

The Lumbar Spine

The lumbar spine is another casualty of life in the modern world. It suffers from too little activity, too much sitting and slouching, and a lack of awareness of how to care for it. I've probably felt close to 10,000 adult lumbar spines in my years of practice, the vast majority of which were stiff. A stiff spine creates several problems for the lower back. The tendons, ligaments, and other soft tissues that attach to it can become strained, the spongy discs that sit between the individual bones can get compressed, and the nerves that travel between the bones of the spine can become pinched.

A stiff spine also has a hard time adapting to the forces applied to it when it's asked to work, even when the work is something as simple as bending over to pick up a suitcase or lifting groceries into or out of the car. Even sneezing can cause problems for someone with a very stiff spine! Rather than being dispersed as they would be by a supple spine, the forces applied during these activities move unevenly and concentrate at tense and vulnerable areas. The result can be excessive pressure on one or two discs between the vertebrae. A herniated—or "blown-out"—disc, therefore, is often a disc that was functioning as something of a release valve, a spot where the pressure applied to the stiff and misaligned spine was forced to find an outlet. On a related side note, some lower back muscle spasms may be the result of a valiant attempt by the body to prevent the damage a herniating disc can do to the vital spinal cord. The muscles "lock down" to prevent further injury—stopping you in your tracks!

SELF TEST: HOW TIGHT IS YOUR LOWER BACK?

A simple test to see if you have a tight lower back is to lie on your stomach and go up onto your elbows, a position known as the "TV watching position" or, in yoga, the "sphinx pose." If this position is hard on your lower back after 30 seconds or less—if it feels at all uncomfortable—your psoas muscles are likely tight and your lumbar spine is stiff.

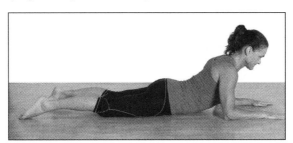

Note: If you've been diagnosed with lumbar spinal stenosis, a herniated disc, or other degenerative disease, you can probably assume your lower back is tight. If you want to try the test anyway, just lie on your stomach without coming up onto your elbows, and stop if it becomes painful!

Fortunately, the movement exercises at the end of this chapter are designed to restore the lower back to health, and the information on habit modification in Chapter Six and seeking help from an outside practitioner in Chapter Seven will help you maintain that health.

Sacroiliac Strain & Lower Back Pain

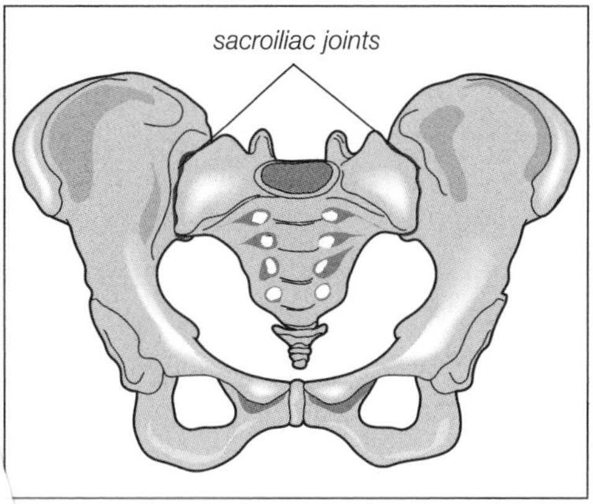

Though not typically as debilitating as the more common causes of lower back pain, strain of the sacroiliac joint(s) is the next most frequently occurring precipitator of the lower back pain cases I see in my office. The ability to locate the exact spot of discomfort is one of the distinguishing features of sacroiliac strain, as is the dull toothachey nature of the pain. The sacroiliac joints are on both sides of the sacrum, which sits at the bottom of the spine, and they connect the sacrum pelvis (figure 4-6). Like all joints of th iliac joints are fluid-fill positionir

Without p a good chance that they'll eventually become irr

In order to fu better acquainted with a marvel of architecture a

Figure 4-6

It's no surprise acred." Long ago, the Greeks understood th re. The Romans, in fact, are purported to ha g it, their use of a "keystone" at the top of an e, triangular sacrum.

The sacrum can be de nt link between the upper and lower halves of the nd hips, which influence your pelvis, which wraps ues, creating the sacroiliac joints. From above, youl oulders, which influence your spine, which descends and con ne top. It's no accident that the meeting spot of the upper and lower sectio ody is the famous and troubled L5-S1 area, which is revealed as a hot spot in so many lower back MRIs.

The sacrum, therefore, is an important and vulnerable bone as it attempts to create harmony between what can often be described as two competing halves of the human frame. And when you combine the pressures exerted on that sacral meeting place, the general lack of varied activity of life in the modern world (joints require a lot of movement to remain healthy), and the predominance of sitting (putting pressure on the bone itself—especially if you're slouching), you can understand just how very at-risk the sacroiliac joints are.

Common Causes of Sacroiliac Strain & Lower Back Pain

One of the happiest events in many women's lives is also one of the most frequent causes of sacroiliac strain: childbirth or, more specifically, giving birth while lying on the back. This delivery position can put pressure on the looser-than-normal (due to a hormone of pregnancy) sacroiliac joints, and many women suffering from lower back pain can clearly trace the origin of their pain to pregnancy and delivery. Other common sources for sacroiliac strain include:

1. Any sort of misstep, such as stepping off a curb by surprise, stepping into a pothole, or missing a step on a staircase, all of which can send a jolt up the leg, shifting the pelvis and sacrum asymmetrically.

2. Bending and twisting simultaneously, as you do when you put a package in the car.

3. Landing on one leg after a jump or a fall.

4. Tilting your pelvis forcefully, like you might do when pressing on a shovel with your foot while digging in the garden.

5. Certain yoga positions held too long.

6. Falling backward onto the sacrum or tailbone.

7. Automobile accidents.

The Added Problem of a Big Belly

Being overweight, especially if it involves having a big belly, creates unique challenges that frequently result in chronic lower back pain and problems. Sometimes, of course, you don't even need to be overweight to suffer from the problems that come from having a big belly; it's a rare woman who doesn't have back pain at some point during the later stages of pregnancy.

The weight of gravity is designed to go through the human body and be accommodated at certain specific areas of its frame. In the lower back, most of that weight is supported by the lumbar spine, which relieves the surrounding muscles and other soft tissues from doing extra, unnecessary work. If you change your body's design, however, by being overweight in general and having a big belly in particular—or by being pregnant—you'll shift the location of the center of gravity and change the places in the lower back where the forces of gravity are being supported, ultimately causing tension, strain, and pain.

The end result is an inherently unstable condition that forces the body to take precautionary action in order to avoid possible disaster. Of all the potential problems, perhaps the most serious is the slipping forward of the lumbar vertebrae, a condition known as spondylolisthesis, which can lead to pinched nerves and a damaged spinal cord. To stabilize the spine and halt any dangerous forward movement of the vertebra, the muscles, tendons, and ligaments of the lower back become taut—like the guy wires of a tent that tighten in order to stabilize the poles.

THE SPINE AS TENT POLE

Imagine your spine as the stabilizing pole at the center of a large circus tent. Like your spine, the tent pole was designed to stand upright and balanced, both bearing and equally distributing the weight of the tent around it. But now let's say one of the circus elephants outside the tent wanders over and manages to sit on one of the tent's outer edges. In response to the stress of the uneven load, the pole is forced to bend as it struggles to keep the tent from collapsing. This not only places a lot of stress on the pole, it also creates a lot of tension in the guy wires, those ropes attached to the stakes placed around the perimeter of the tent to further support it and prevent it from falling down. In this analogy, the elephant sitting on the tent represents a larger-than-normal belly placing uneven stress on your spine—the tent pole—and your lower back muscles and supporting ligaments are the guy wires that are under constant tension, assisting your spine in its attempt to stay upright.

Sciatica & Piriformis Syndrome

The sciatic nerve is the largest nerve in the human body. It originates in the lumbar spine and travels through the buttocks on its way down the legs to the feet. Sciatica is the term given for pain, numbness, or tingling radiating down one or, rarely, both legs as a result of pressure on the sciatic nerve or its roots. If it progresses, weakness in the affected leg or foot may also be experienced.

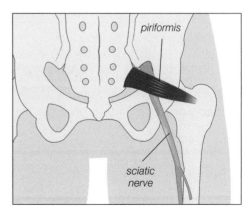

Figure 4-7. Rear view of pelvis

Two well-known causes of sciatica are: 1) a herniated disc pressing on the spinal roots, and 2) spinal stenosis—an abnormal narrowing in the spinal canal that restricts nerves. The sciatic nerve can also get pinched, however, as it travels away from the spine, and this, too, causes problems. When the piriformis (pronounced *peer-ih-form-us*) muscle, located deep in the butt area, becomes tight or enlarged, it's apt to press on the sciatic nerve as it passes by (figure 4-7).

This problem, referred to as piriformis syndrome, is a much more common cause of sciatica than most patients, and their doctors, realize. In fact, while some doctors still doubt its very existence:

> *The prestigious Institute for Spinal Disorders at Cedars Sinai Medical Center in Los Angeles performed advanced studies on 239 patients with sciatica who had failed to improve with traditional treatment. After advanced imaging of the nerves and muscles, 67% of the patients were rediagnosed as having piriformis syndrome.*[13]

Another study sheds further light on the source and treatment of sciatic pain:

> *The neurosurgical department at Leiden University in the Netherlands undertook a systematic review of the literature to determine the effectiveness of surgery in patients with sciatica due to a lumbar disc herniation versus conservative treatments. They concluded that there were no significant differences between the surgical and conservatively managed groups after one and two years.*[14]

It's important to note that when the source of sciatica was determined to be pressure from a herniated lumbar disc, *surgical intervention did not produce any better results than more conservative treatment in the long run*. This could mean that either the problem was initially incorrectly diagnosed as resulting from a herniated lumbar disc when it was actually piriformis syndrome, or that disc herniations can be effectively treated with conservative treatment, or both.

The reason that piriformis syndrome is so difficult for the modern medical community to recognize is that they usually limit their diagnostic approach to sciatica to the viewing of the spine through X-rays and MRIs. Broadening the diagnostic approach by examining the muscles as well as the spine, and by asking the right questions, yields additional information and a greater likelihood of an accurate diagnosis. Using this broader approach, the findings that would lead to the diagnosis of piriformis syndrome include:

1. Patients report that sciatic symptoms worsen when sitting—certain car seats seem to be particularly aggravating—as pressure on the butt can irritate the muscle and nerve.

2. Patients display obvious tension and discomfort when they perform the piriformis muscle stretch.

3. The patient practically jumps off the table from pain when the practitioner presses on the piriformis muscle on the involved side.

4. A week or two of heat or ice, stretching, and hands-on treatment usually significantly improve the patient's symptoms.

Arthritis, Disc Disease, Spinal Stenosis, & Other Scapegoats

If you've read the chapter to this point, you've discovered that the cause of most cases of lower back pain is misalignment and tension, whose two main targets are the muscles and spine of the lower back. So what do we make of the conditions most commonly blamed for people's lower back pain—arthritis, degenerative disease, spinal stenosis, disc bulges, and herniations?

Before we talk about those common scapegoats, let's first look at the means through with which they're discovered—the modern medical doctor's best friends—X-rays and MRIs.

X-RAYS AND MRIS

X-rays and MRIs are wonderful tools if you're looking for fractures, serious spinal impingements, tumors, or other systemic diseases, but they have very limited use for the average case of lower back pain because they:

1. Cannot take into consideration that the source of the problem may be distant from the site of the patient's pain ("referred pain");

2. Can and do reveal things that may seem to be, but are not, the real cause of pain (since pain-free people often have the same findings);

3. Can be and are occasionally misread and misinterpreted by physicians.

These are significant shortcomings, so let's examine them further. It's well known in medicine that pain can radiate to a joint above and a joint below the actual problem area, and quite possibly even further. Hip dysfunction, for example, can cause pain to radiate to the lower back above, and/or to the knee below. So even though your hip is the real problem, your lower back is likely thought to be the source of the problem and an MRI of that area is ordered. Not only can't the MRI of your lower back inform the physician that the problem is in your hip, but it will also more than likely reveal something in the lumbar spine that will be erroneously labeled as the cause of your suffering!

Well, you may say, if an X-ray or MRI shows arthritis or a bulging disc in my lower back, then surely that must be relevant, or at least it must represent another source of my pain. As hard as it may be to believe, this assumption simply isn't true. If it were, we wouldn't find degenerative conditions in people who have no current or past history of back pain. But a lot of research shows that plenty of pain-free people *do* have degenerative conditions.

As reported in the 1994 New England Journal of Medicine, *researchers performed MRI examinations on 98 pain-free volunteers and discovered that 52% had disc bulges and 27% had disc protrusions (38% of them had these findings at more than one disc level!). Additionally, 8% to 19% of the asymptomatic subjects also had MRI findings of facet arthropathy, annular defects, and Schmorl's nodes. This prompted the authors to conclude that "given the high prevalence of these findings...the discovery by MRI of bulges and protrusions in people with lower back pain may frequently be coincidental."[15]*

Spinal stenosis studies have demonstrated that the results of these imaging studies frequently don't differentiate symptomatic people from those without symptoms, meaning that significant percentages of people with no pain at all also have findings consistent with spinal stenosis on MRIs.[16, 17] This fact prompted a University of Michigan research team to conclude that "radiographic findings alone are insufficient to justify treatment for spinal stenosis."[18]

The final point about X-rays and MRIs is probably obvious but still bears mention. X-rays and MRIs must be taken by technicians and read by physicians, meaning the skills of the people taking the image and reading the film play an important role in diagnosis. And even the most skilled people make mistakes. Add to these realities the fact that the quality of the image is also an important factor in the accuracy of a diagnosis, and you can see how much room for error exists.

The True Significance of Radiologic Findings

The true significance of common radiologic findings like arthritis, disc disease, and stenosis, even when they're relevant to the patient's complaint, is that to some extent they reflect the level of tension and misalignment in the body. The degenerative changes seen on X-rays and MRIs are typically the end result of some combination of the molding of the human body from poor postural habits and from slips, falls, and other trauma.

To address the findings of arthritis, disc problems, and stenosis as most physicians do misses the point and ignores the cause. Reduce the tension in the body, creating more "space" and mobility in the frame, and not only will pain ease but over time the body in its wisdom and capacity to heal can actually begin to remove the degeneration by laying down new cartilage, reabsorbing disc bulges, and remodeling bone. Of course, not every case of degeneration is reversible, but my patients frequently discover that releasing the tension within the spine and surrounding soft tissues through stretching, strengthening, range-of-motion exercises, postural improvements, and hands-on body work eliminates or significantly reduces their back pain while their radiologic findings may or may not live on.

In short, given an improved environment, the body can and will, by design, attempt to self-correct. But we must give it a chance by addressing the cause and not focusing on the results found on two-dimensional films and lab reports.

Surgery or Conservative Therapy?

Unfortunately, invasive approaches to lower back pain—surgery, for instance—not only often fail to produce better results than conservative ones do, but also carry potentially devastating side effects. Still, approximately 1.2 million people elect to have spinal surgery, including 300,000 spinal fusions, every year.[19] Though there are times when invasive procedures may be a necessary last resort, it's important to remember that they focus on the signs of the molding process—the narrowing spaces and bulging and herniated discs—and justify their need on diagnoses obtained from X-rays and MRIs, which, as we have seen, aren't always reliable. A better method of addressing lower back pain, therefore, is a conservative approach that addresses the molded, tense body itself and ignores—at least temporarily—those radiographic findings. So what do the studies show?

> A Norwegian orthopedic study, as reported in the journal Spine, compared the effectiveness of lumbar fusion surgery followed by physical therapy with the non-surgical approach of exercise and education on the use of the back in patients with lower back pain lasting more than one year and evidence of lumbar disc degeneration on radiographic examination. They concluded that those patients who skipped surgery for conservative treatment did equally well.[20]

> An English orthopedic group reported a similar finding in the British Medical Journal, concluding that "no clear evidence emerged that primary spinal fusion surgery was any more beneficial than intensive rehabilitation" for chronic lower back pain.[21]

It's also possible that some of the surgeries that are successful actually owe their success to the months of physical therapy that inevitably follow back surgery. So why not skip the surgery altogether and go right to therapy, supervised by an expert, or done at home?

Let's Get Started

As mentioned in the previous chapter, I often compare a tight, molded back to a bucket full to the brim with water, where any added stress becomes another drop causing it to overflow. Releasing tension from the body is like removing some of the water from the bucket, which as a result can now accept more without spilling over. So let's move on to the treatment section so you can begin to empty your lower back bucket, experience pain relief, and prevent future problems from occurring.

ZONE 2 PROGRAM: The Lower Back

STRETCHING		
EXERCISE	REP	DURATION
Psoas, page 53	1	:30
Piriformis in a Chair (both sides), page 55	1	:30 x 2
Gluteals (both sides), page 56	1	:30 x 2
STRENGTHENING		
Spinal Extensors, page 57	1	:30
RANGE-OF-MOTION		
Flexion/Extension, page 59	1	:30
Side Bending, page 60	1	:30
Rotation, page 61	1	:30
Total time of daily workout		4:30

The key to both curing and preventing lower back pain and problems is to do some targeted exercises to unwrap it from the imaginary ball placed in front of it. The stretching exercises will *loosen* the short and tight lower back flexors, and the strengthening exercises will *strengthen* the overly stretched and weak back extensors. The range-of-motion exercises will help to *lubricate* and *release tension* in the lumbar spine. Only then is there a chance for the lower back to return to a state of improved alignment and flexibility, allowing blood flow to improve, inflammation and waste products to be removed, nerves to travel unimpeded, muscles and other soft tissues to return to their original length and tone, and bulging discs to become reabsorbed.

NOTE: Make sure you've read Chapter Two (page 14) for important general information about movement.

Hold all stretches a minimum of 30 seconds and do each at least once.

Psoas Stretch

In some ways this is the most important lower back stretch you can do. We spend most of our day sitting or bending forward, wrapped around that imaginary ball in our lap, and have few opportunities to counteract this forward positioning with natural backward-bending activities. This stretch puts the imaginary ball behind you, in a manner of speaking. If you've ever done yoga, you'll recognize these stretches as sphinx and upward-facing dog, or cobra, two staple yoga poses.

There's a lot of fear about bending backward, especially where spinal stenosis or other degenerative conditions are present, but the psoas needs to be stretched. As usual, go slowly, stop if it hurts, and seek guidance for other variations of this stretch if necessary.

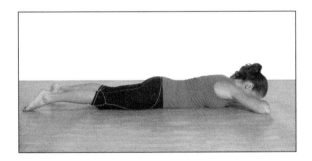

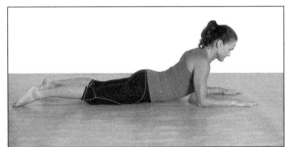

1. Lying flat on your stomach, head resting on the backs of your crossed hands, relax your belly and feel the natural curve of your lower back. For many of my older patients, this is enough of a stretch, for a week or two at least, as they'll feel tension in the lower back region without going any farther.

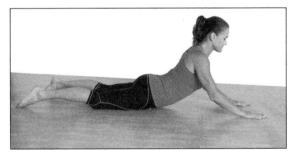

2. If lying face down as above doesn't provide a stretch and your lower back is in pretty good shape, then try coming up onto your elbows (the sphinx pose in yoga) or the palms of your hands (the cobra yoga pose). Just remember: It's more important to relax the belly and let the lower back stretch gently than it is to try to go up higher.

ALTERNATE VERSION: A much less effective (because the muscles are not as relaxed when standing and the stretch is not held long enough) but more convenient way to stretch the hip flexors is to bend backward while standing. This is a good postural exercise and helps to counteract all of the sitting and forward bending we do throughout the day.

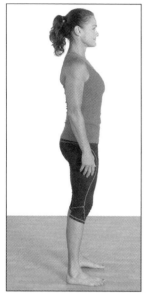
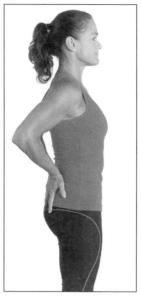
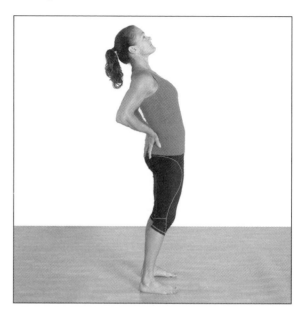

1. Stand upright, feet about shoulder-width apart. Place your hands on your lower back, fingers pointing back and down.

2. Bend backward as far as you comfortably can, using your hands for support.

Hold this position for 2–3 seconds and return to the upright position. Repeat throughout the day to break the grip of forward bending.

Piriformis Stretch in a Chair

The piriformis muscle needs to be stretched to reduce the potential pressure it can put on the sciatic nerve (a problem called piriformis syndrome) and to assist in releasing tension in the sacroiliac joints.

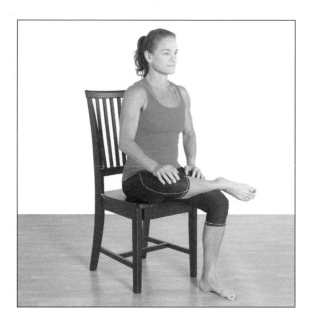 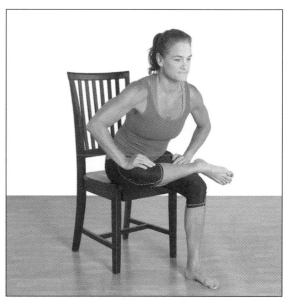

1. Sitting in a chair, bring your right ankle to rest on top of your left thigh, just above the knee.

2. Gently hinge at the waist, leaning your upper body forward until you feel a stretch in your thigh/butt area. Make sure to keep your upper and lower back straight rather than letting it round. In other words, don't slump!

Repeat on the other side.

Gluteal Stretch

The gluteal muscles are very powerful and play a major role in the positioning and functioning of the pelvis and lower back and therefore play a major role in the health of the region.

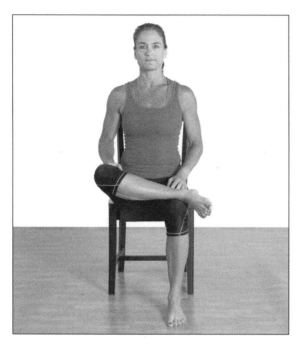

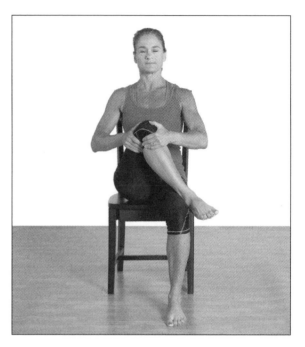

1. Sitting in a chair, bring your right ankle to rest on top of your left thigh, just above the knee.

2. Reaching with both hands, grab your right knee and, leaving the right ankle in place— resting on the left thigh—bring your right knee up and over across your stomach and toward your left side until you feel a stretch in the thigh/butt area. Think in terms of bringing your right knee over to touch your left shoulder without dipping your shoulder down. You won't actually be able to touch your shoulder, of course, unless you lower your shoulder or move your right ankle from your left thigh (don't do either of these), but the idea of moving *toward* your left shoulder may help you.

Repeat on the other side.

Hold all exercises a minimum of 30 seconds and do each at least once.

Spinal Extensors

As mentioned earlier, studies have revealed the extensor muscles of the back to be weak—the result of too much sitting and other common habits—in people with chronic lower back pain. These same studies have shown that strengthening the extensors results in reduced pain and dysfunction. The strengthening exercise I recommend puts minimal pressure on the spine—important if you have a history of a lower back injury—while still challenging the muscles to get stronger.

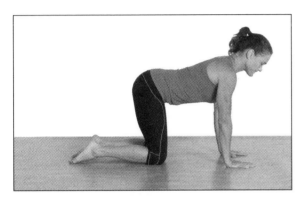

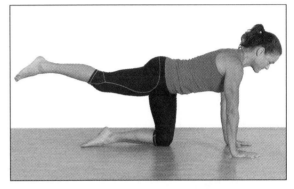

1. Start from your hands and knees in a flat-back tabletop position, with knees hip-width apart and hands shoulder-width apart.

2. Engage your abdominal muscles by pulling your belly toward your spine. While keeping your neck and back in a straight line (look straight down, and don't arch your lower back), extend your right leg straight back until it's parallel to the floor.

Hold for as long as you can maintain good form, up to 10 seconds. Repeat 3 times with each leg, 3 days a week, with a day or two of rest in between.

NOTE: If your back is in good shape and you find the above exercise to be easy, replace it with one from below.

MORE CHALLENGING VERSION: Try extending the opposite arm out in front of you at the same time as you're extending the leg behind. Both the leg and arm should point out straight, parallel to the floor. Repeat the exercise with the other arm and leg.

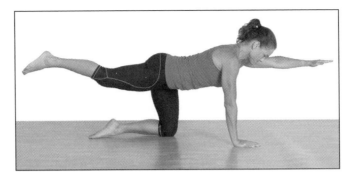

MOST CHALLENGING VERSION: If you find the above strengthening exercises too easy, and you have no history of lower back problems, try this version—known as the prone back extension— which puts more pressure on the spine but works the muscles harder than the above versions.

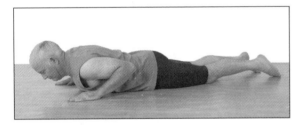

1. Lie facedown on the floor with your hands beneath your shoulders. Keep your head and neck relaxed by looking at the floor just an inch or two in front of you.

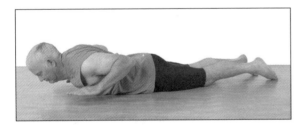

2. You're not actually going to be using your hands and arms to push up, so before you begin the exercise, pull your hands up off the floor—keeping your arms and elbows tight against your sides—so that they hover a few inches off the floor.

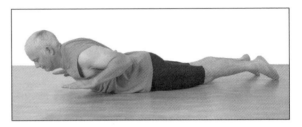

3. Now do a "push-up" by lifting just your chest up a few inches off the floor, and immediately lowering it to the starting position.

Do as many as you comfortably can, working up to 10 to 12 total, 3 days a week, with a day or two of rest in between.

Perform range-of-motion maneuvers a minimum of 30 seconds and do each at least once.

Flexion/Extension

It's important to move the lumbar spine regularly in all three of its planes of motion in order to keep it pliable. You don't need to hold these positions. Just move gently—and slowly—in one direction until you feel resistance, and then move in the opposite direction. Repeat several times until you begin to feel a little looser. Small amounts of movement are all that is required. This version of flexion/ extension is called "cat and cow" in yoga.

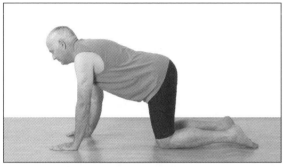

1. Starting from your hands and knees in a flat-back tabletop position.

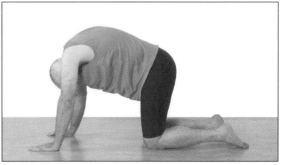

3. Once you reach your stopping point (don't push), slowly exhale while rounding your back, contracting your stomach, and dropping your head.

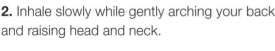

2. Inhale slowly while gently arching your back and raising head and neck.

MODIFICATION: This can also be done standing by simply alter-nating between gentle forward hunching and backward arching.

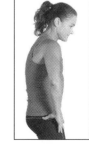
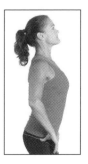

Side Bending

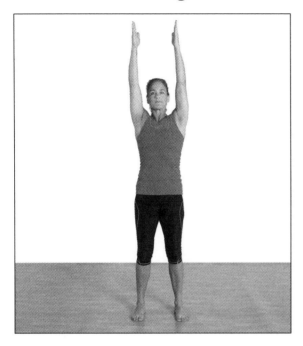

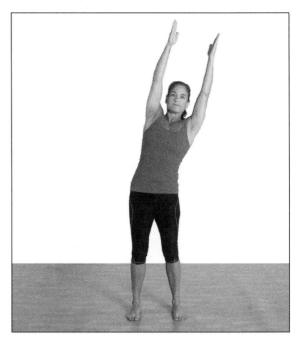

1. Stand or sit with your torso tall and arms extended overhead.

2. Keeping your arms straight, lean your upper body—from your waist—to the right, as far as you can comfortably go. When you've reached that point, move back to the center starting position, and then immediately proceed to the left-leaning position.

MODIFICATION: If you have trouble reaching your arms overhead due to shoulder restriction, do the exercise with your arms at your sides, sliding your hands one-at-a-time down each thigh to accomplish the side bending.

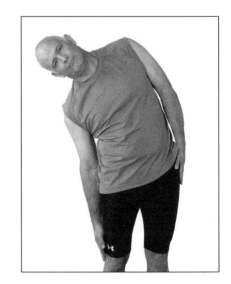

Rotation

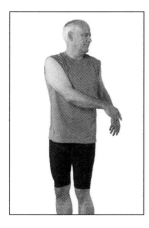 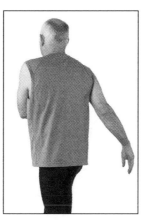

1–2. With your arms relaxed at your sides, gently rotate your upper body around to the right and left, in a rhythmic motion, until you feel resistance. Don't rush it and your spine will get a nice rotary stretch.

CHAPTER FIVE
Zone 3: The Lower Body
Hips, Knees, & Feet

Natural forces within us are the true healers of disease.

—Hippocrates

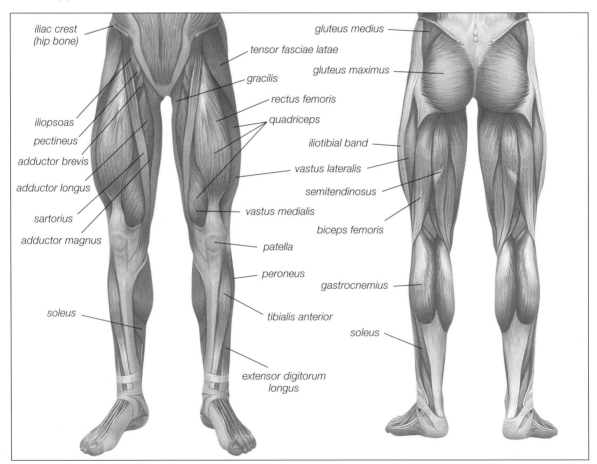

iliac crest (hip bone)

gluteus medius

tensor fasciae latae

gluteus maximus

gracilis

rectus femoris

iliopsoas

quadriceps

pectineus

iliotibial band

adductor brevis

vastus lateralis

adductor longus

semitendinosus

sartorius

vastus medialis

adductor magnus

biceps femoris

patella

peroneus

gastrocnemius

soleus

tibialis anterior

soleus

extensor digitorum longus

Zone 3 consists of the hips, the knees, and the feet, the areas of the lower body that cause people the most trouble and pain. Working together, they perform two very important jobs: bearing the weight of the body and moving it. Partially as a result of the demands of these two critical functions, the most chronic and debilitating musculoskeletal problems come from this region.

As with zones 1 and 2, it's important to check in with your family physician for an "official" medical diagnosis for your pain and other symptoms. But also as with the other zones, modern medicine has almost no role to play in the average case of lower body pain. Unless you have one of the rare and more serious conditions sometimes associated with hip or knee pain, like a joint infection, all the modern medical doctor can do is offer you a prescription for anti-inflammatories and painkillers, or perform invasive procedures. Neither of these responses is apt to address the real issue, and both have potentially harmful side effects.

One Million Replacements & Counting

Hip, knee, and foot pain are very common complaints in today's world. Difficulties with the lower body generally become more common and more serious as people reach their middle and later years, though it's possible for a younger person to have pain and problems, especially if there's a history of trauma. Hips and knees are so problematic that there are upward of 1,000,000 hip and knee replacement surgeries performed in the United States every year, and that number, according to the American Association of Hip and Knee Surgeons, is expected to more than triple by 2030.

In case you were going to argue that swapping out joints is an acceptable solution to the problems that plague so many, I would counter that not only is avoiding major surgery and its complications something to be strongly desired, but also that the outcomes of such joint replacement surgeries are not always rosy. A recent study cited in the *British Journal of Medicine* reviewed published data regarding patient reports of pain from three months to five years following total hip or knee replacements. The range of people reporting unfavorable long-term pain outcomes was 7% to 23% after hip replacements and 10% to 34% after knee replacements.[22] These are significant numbers, and while there are times when joint replacements are necessary and helpful, they reflect a complex problem that deserves an alternative solution.

Molded & Misaligned

Most pain in the hip and knee areas comes from problems in and around the joints themselves. A joint is nothing more than the coming together of two different parts of the body. The hip is the meeting place of the pelvis and the thigh, and the knee is where the thigh and leg (anatomically speaking, the leg is the part of the limb between the ankle and the knee) connect. As with all parts of the body, joints require the proper orientation and alignment of the two areas that are meeting in order to be functional and pain-free. In other words, if the pelvis and thigh are improperly aligned, the hip joint will eventually suffer; if the thigh and leg are improperly aligned, the knee joint will suffer. And since you cannot move one end of a bone without also moving its other end, a foot, ankle, knee, or hip that's misaligned will have a domino effect on the whole lower extremity, not to mention all the way on up through the body.

In the vast majority of people, the body gets gripped over time by our work and play habits, creating a mold or pattern where one or both of the lower limbs become misaligned, causing it (or them) to have to bear the weight of the body and move it along in ways it wasn't designed to do. This is no less than a recipe for disaster. *You cannot change the design or position of something in the human body without changing the way it functions*. Think of alignment as it relates to a car. If the front end is misaligned, the tires will wear out unevenly, and more quickly, than they would if the alignment was true. Similarly, even the slightest change in the alignment of the lower limbs puts stress on places that weren't intended to receive it, which is why it can take surprisingly little activity to irritate and inflame our lower limbs and joints as we get older. Think, in comparison, of the way young (well-aligned) children can play at the park all day, every day, without a problem.

In the hips and knees, the misalignment sets the stage for the acute problems of tendinitis and bursitis. Worse still, years of walking with misaligned lower limbs creates muscle weakness and dysfunction, arthritis, meniscal tears, degenerative changes, and a loss of joint space resulting in "bone-on-bone" knee and hip joint conditions. In the feet, the end result of years spent moving incorrectly is the formation of bunions, pain between the toes (neuromas), and pain on the bottom of the feet (plantar fasciitis), among other problems.

The end result of simply getting up, sitting down, and walking throughout the day with lower body misalignment is that the effects of even the slightest amounts of asymmetry and tension becomes amplified, leading to premature and ongoing pain and problems. This isn't to say that we shouldn't move, but that we need to be aware of *how* we move and make every effort to do so correctly—to get back on the right path, as I say to my patients.

A PATH IN THE GRASS

Imagine a front yard with a well-tended lawn and an elegantly designed stone path that leads from the driveway to your front door. One day you take a shortcut across the lawn rather than walking on the path. For a while, the lawn puts up with your behavior and things seem fine. Eventually, however, a wear pattern begins to show up. The dirt below is exposed and an earthen trail reveals the new pattern that's been established by repeatedly walking off the intended path.

In your feet, knees, and hips, the wear patterns from walking improperly are felt as aches and pains and revealed on X-rays as tears, arthritis, degeneration, and eventually as a reduction of the space in the joints. In an attempt to remedy the situation, many of my patients take supplements, like glucosamine, as raw materials to help repair damaged joints. Though this may help, a lack of raw materials is not the real problem and supplying new ones is not the real solution. In our path analogy, it would be like planting grass seed on your worn-out path in the hope that new grass will start to grow even as you're still trampling on it every day. Once you correct your movement and get back on the right path, you'll stop wearing out your joints and then your body will have a chance to repair the damage and heal itself. In other words, the grass will grow back by itself if you stop walking on it!

Common Habits That Compromise the Lower Body

Although the misalignment of the lower limbs can take many forms, the most common one I observe in the bodies of my patients is that of the legs rotating outward, turning more toward the side than straight ahead. This is seen most easily when an individual's feet point more laterally than forward as he or she walks (figure 5-1).

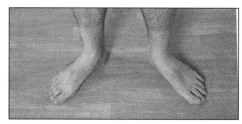

Figure 5-1

Many of the habits and activities that we typically engage in create this outward rotation of the lower limb, which eventually becomes a permanent condition. One of the most common habits is crossing the legs when sitting or lying down, either with one ankle resting upon the opposite thigh, or with both legs crossed at the ankles (figure 5-2). My older patients frequently cross their outstretched legs when they lie face-up on my treatment table. They do this because they're no longer comfortable lying with their legs in proper alignment, and crossing their ankles relieves the tension created when their legs face straight up. Unfortunately, these cross-legged positions, whether sitting up or lying down, only add to the existing misalignment.

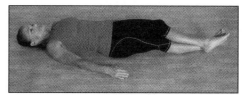

Other habits and activities that create this mold include the natural tendency to point the feet toward the sides when driving a car (especially the right foot on the gas pedal) and sleeping in positions that push the feet laterally, like sleeping on your stomach with one leg hiked

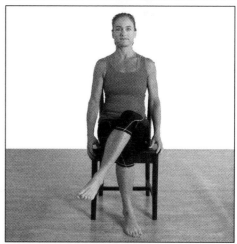

Figure 5-2

up, or on your back with the weight of the covers pushing the feet outward, as if you were a ballet dancer in first position.

As we discussed in Chapter Four, another unfortunate habit that molds the body is too much sitting. Sitting both 1) shortens and weakens the hip flexor muscles (the psoas muscle being the largest and most powerful one) that connect the trunk of the body to the lower limbs, and 2) lengthens and weakens the butt muscles, or gluteals (gluteus maximus, medius, and mimimus). As we'll discuss in the next section, one of the consequences to these muscles of so much sitting is the further rotation of the lower limbs, adding to the problems of the hips, knees, and feet.

The Main Players in the Misalignment of the Lower Limbs

The two groups of muscles that are most affected by the molding process of the lower limbs are the hip rotators and flexors. Not surprisingly, these are also the most consistently tight and, when pressed upon, the tenderest muscles in the lower bodies of my patients.

The Hip Rotators

The hip rotators are the very important muscles responsible for turning the lower limbs inward or outward. Though some people walk pigeon-toed, where the feet turn inward, by far the more common pattern I observe is the "duck walk," where the feet point noticeably outward (figure 5-1). This is primarily the result of the external rotators of the hip getting shorter and tighter as a result of those habits we've just discussed. Although we'll focus on the more-common problems of the external rotators, the stretches at the end of this section are designed to resolve tension in both the internal and external rotators. In other words, they're for pigeons and ducks alike.

The foot, knee, and hip joints were designed to move in one basic direction—forward—following a mostly forward-pointing foot (with just a bit of external rotation). If instead one or both of the feet are pointing too far to the side, the joints will be forced to add extra rotation to their back-and-forth movement in order to accommodate. This rotating, or grinding, action creates tremendous pressure, or torque, inside the joints and on the surrounding soft tissues, resulting in serious damage over time (figure 5-3).

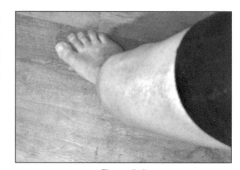

Figure 5-3

One of the main external rotators of the hip, the piriformis muscle, originates at the side of the sacrum (the bone at the bottom of the spine) and ends at the thigh bone, or femur, near the hip joint. Tension in this muscle can therefore create painful problems for the hip as well as for the lower back. Not surprisingly, lower back pain and hip pain are frequently present together in the same patient. In addition, piriformis muscle tension can also create piriformis syndrome, a condition where the muscle presses on the sciatic nerve as it passes by, creating radiating pain or numbness down the leg (see "Sciatica and Piriformis Syndrome" on page 47 for a full discussion).

As an added problem, I frequently discover a significant asymmetry or imbalance in the hip rotators from one side of the body to the other. This is most likely the result of such habits as always having the right foot turned out on the gas pedal, favoring one sleep position over others, or tending to favor one leg crossed over the other. Alone, tension in the hip rotator muscles is bad enough, but asymmetry from one side to the other creates a whole new set of challenges for the body to cope with.

SELF-TEST: HOW SYMMETRIC ARE YOUR HIPS?

To test your own hip-muscle symmetry, sit in a chair and alternately place each ankle on top of the opposite thigh, just above the knee. Is one leg easier to cross than the other? Are the positions of the resting crossed legs similar to each other, or is one leg more parallel or perpendicular to the ground than the other?

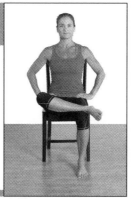
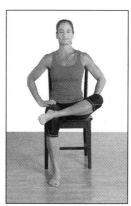

On a final, slightly more technical note, the hip rotators also have the very important job of helping to steady the hip joint by keeping the thigh bone properly situated in the pelvic joint capsule, or acetabulum. This means that the proper length, tone, and symmetry of these rotator muscles play an important role in the general positioning, and therefore the health and stability, of the hip joint itself.

The Hip Flexors

The hip flexors are powerful core muscles connecting the trunk of the body to the lower limbs. The primary hip flexors are the psoas muscles, which allow you to lift your thighs toward your trunk or bend your trunk forward toward your thighs. These are also the muscles that frequently strain or go into spasm, causing debilitating lower back pain when you lift up a child, bend and twist to put a package in the car, or even just sneeze!

As discussed in detail in Chapter Four, too much sitting is the main nemesis of the hip flexors, as they eventually become shorter, tighter, and weaker. Compounding the problem is the fact that as adults we rarely bend backward to stretch these muscles as we did naturally when we were children during gym class, on the playground, or participating in a sport. Too much sitting and not enough stretching eventually leads not only to back pain but also to joint problems in the lower body.

This happens for two main reasons. First, like the hip rotators, the hip flexors also help to stabilize and steady the hip joint itself. Tension, misalignment, and asymmetry in the psoas muscles, therefore, can compromise the position and proper functioning of the hip joint, causing the aches, pains, and the degenerative problems that follow. Second, in addition to flexing the hip, the psoas muscles (in addition to the piriformis muscles) also function as external rotators of the lower limbs. Tension in these muscles, therefore, can cause the legs to further externally rotate, contributing to the misalignment, pain, and problems in the hip, knee, and foot.

Eventually, the hip flexors can become so tight that we may find that we can't even stand or walk fully erect anymore and are forced to take short, bent-over, shuffling steps with feet pointed outward. We've all seen elderly people like this (figure 5-4) and, although the bent-over shuffle represents an extreme situation, subtler versions of this painful posture and gait are quite common.

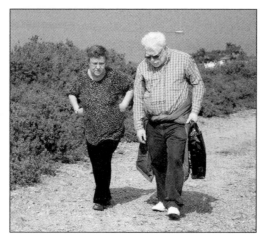

Figure 5-4

Individual Components of Zone 3

Now that you have a general idea of the grip on the lower body that our habits create, let's take a look at some of the ways it affects the individual components of Zone 3 and what some of the research studies reveal:

Hip Pain

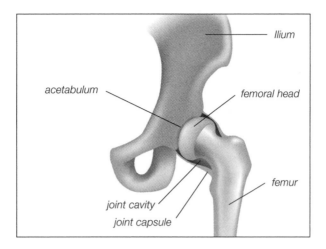

- Hip pain is commonly located deep in the hip area itself, in the front of the thigh, or in the groin area, but can be felt in the buttock, lower back, or other areas of the thigh. The wide and varied distribution of pain can make an accurate diagnosis difficult.

- In its early stages, problems of the hip create intermittent pain typically experienced as dull and achy. Joint stiffness, common when first getting out of bed or after prolonged sitting, improves with movement.

- As hip dysfunction progresses, the range of motion of the joint becomes more limited and the pain becomes more constant, sharper, and more debilitating, and worsens with walking and other types of physical activity.

Radiological findings of arthritis, degenerative disease, tears of the labrum, bursitis, and tendinitis (also known as "trochanteric pain syndrome") are too frequently diagnosed as the cause of a patient's hip pain. These radiological findings are easy targets because they appear on many X-rays and MRIs of adults. The fact is that there's ample evidence to demonstrate that these same findings appear on the X-rays and MRIs of people who have no complaints of pain at all. For example:

A study conducted by the Steadman Philippon Research Institute's Center for Outcomes-based Orthopedic Research recruited 45 volunteers, the average age being 37.8 years, with no history of hip pain, injury, or surgery to undergo MRI scans of the hip. The results of the MRIs revealed: labral tears in 69% of the volunteers, chondral defects in 24%, subchondral cysts in 16%, and osseous bumps in 20%, among other abnormalities reported.[23]

The Department of Radiology at the University of Wisconsin School of Medicine and Public Health retrospectively reviewed MRIs of 240 hips of people without pain and discovered that 88% revealed abnormalities, leading the authors to conclude that "detection of these abnormalities on MRI is a poor predictor of trochanteric pain syndrome as these findings are present in a high percentage of patients without trochanteric pain."[24]

Knee Pain

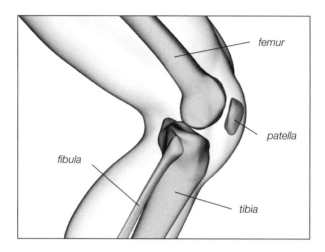

- Knee pain is typically dull and achy and worsens with walking, stair-climbing, and other forms of physical activity. The pain can be located anywhere around the knee and can radiate to the hip or ankle.

- As it progresses, knee dysfunction can create stiffness after prolonged sitting, swelling and warmth around the joint, and pain at rest.

- Popping sounds or grinding sensations when bending the knee, as well as joint instability, are frequently the result of a misaligned knee cap and weak thigh muscles.

Radiological findings of arthritis, degenerative disease, and tears of the meniscus are too frequently diagnosed as the cause of a patient's knee pain. As with the hip and other areas, radiologic findings like these become easy targets because they appear on many X-rays and MRIs of adults, even while ample evidence exists demonstrating that the same findings appear on the films of people with no pain at all. For example:

To examine the link between meniscal tears and pain, the Boston University Medical Center's Department of Orthopedics performed MRIs on 49 people with no complaints of knee pain and discovered that 76% of them had medial or lateral meniscal tears, calling them "a very common finding in the asymptomatic subjects."[25]

Looking at the association between knee pain and osteoarthritis, data from the National Health and Nutrition Survey (NHANES I) was analyzed by the Harvard Medical School Division on Aging, which revealed that of 319 subjects with evidence of stage 2-4 knee osteoarthritis on X-rays, only 47% of them reported knee pain.[26] (Stages 2-4 osteoarthritis describe mild to severe conditions.)

After a systematic search and summary of the literature, an arthritis research group at Keele University in the United Kingdom concluded that knee osteoarthritis reported on X-rays is "an imprecise guide to the likelihood that knee pain or disability will be present."[27]

The flip side of the coin, as you might have suspected, is that studies also reveal that many people who complain of knee pain, some of whom are actually diagnosed as having knee arthritis by their physician, actually have no sign of significant arthritis on X-rays.

A study done in coordination with the Harvard Medical School Division on Aging analyzed the data from NHANES I and found that of 1004 subjects complaining of knee pain, only 15% had significant (stage 2-4) knee arthritis on X-ray. This same study found that while 1,762 subjects reported having been diagnosed with arthritis by their physician, only 11% of them actually had stage 2-4 osteoarthritis on X-ray.[28]

Foot Pain

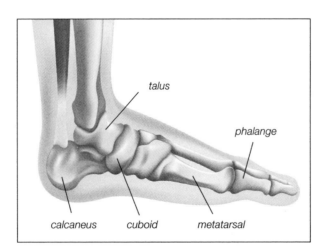

- Foot pain can be dull and annoying but is more frequently sharp and debilitating, especially when weight is placed on it.

- The most common source of foot pain is not acute trauma but the long-term subtle changes to the foot as a result of the many miles logged walking, often incorrectly, in poorly designed footwear on hard and unyielding surfaces.

- Changes to the foot over time typically result in fallen arches, the formation of bunions, strain on the fascia that line the bottom of the foot (plantar fasciitis), pinched nerves between the toes (Morton's neuroma), compound fractures, and muscle cramps. All of these problems are structural in nature and can be prevented and improved with conservative care—stretching and range-of-motion exercises, hands-on work, and improved mechanics of walking.

The Foundation of the Body—More About the Feet

The feet are the foundation of the body and our sole contact with the earth as we move about in the world. They are marvels of architecture and engineering, containing some 26 bones, 33 joints, and more than 100 muscles, tendons, and ligaments. The foot must be strong enough to support the weight of the body yet flexible enough to move it along on a variety of different surfaces.

These amazing physical structures were designed to walk barefoot on the yielding ground. First, the hard-hitting heel sinks down into the earth, which cushions the impact of contact. The arch is then perfectly supported as the earth essentially rises up to meet it. Finally, the ball of the foot and the toes press into a ground that gives way yet provides enough resistance to propel the foot forward.

In contrast, the hard, unyielding, and punishing surfaces of the modern world—pavement, concrete, wood, and tile—give no cushioning or support to the feet. When you consider that studies show we take an average of 5,000–10,000 steps a day, it becomes obvious why so many people suffer from aches, pains, and problems as they get older. And while modern footwear may absorb some of the shock, it also takes away a lot of the work that the individual muscles of the foot would normally do if the foot was bare, making those muscles weaker and weaker over time and creating all of those foot problems listed above.

SELF-TEST: HOW WEAK ARE YOUR FOOT MUSCLES?

One way to determine how weak the muscles of your feet have become is to see how far you can walk barefoot on the beach—if you're lucky enough to have one near—or, to a lesser extent, on the lawn. Walking on soft surfaces engages all of the muscles of the foot, and most middle-aged and older people will quickly discover that they can't walk very far before their feet begin to cramp and ache.

While a couple of the movement exercises that follow will indirectly exercise the feet, one of the best things you can do to engage the bones, muscles, and soft tissues of the feet, stretching and strengthening them and using them as they were designed to be used, is to spend some time outside walking barefoot on the earth. More about this in Chapter Eight.

Bunions

It has been my observation that a high percentage of the patients who arrive at my office with chronic and recurrent hip or knee pain also have bunions forming on their feet (or have had them removed surgically). While opinions differ as to the origin of bunions, I believe a common cause is years spent walking with misaligned lower limbs.

When the foot strikes the ground from a flared-out position—pointing too far to the side—it lands more on the outer edge of the heel and, as a consequence, must then roll over more toward the inside edge—near the base of the big toe—as it prepares to push-off (figure 5-5). (A forward-facing foot can also excessively roll toward the inside, or pronate, as a result of flat feet.) This creates tremendous pressure and wear and tear on an area—the base of the big toe (not the big toe itself)—that was not designed to handle it. The body, the amazing problem-solver that it is, responds to this misplaced pressure by attempting to grow you a new toe, sort of a sixth toe—or bunion—to push off from.

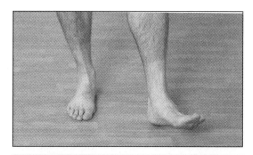
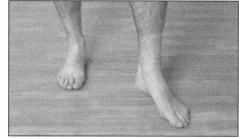

Figure 5-5

The formation of bunions, therefore, often thought of as another body malfunction, is actually another example of the body's attempt to make the best of a bad situation.

To put it another way, bunions are the effects and not the cause of the problem, and therefore although you can remove them, you haven't solved the real problem. As many people have discovered, the removal of their bunions not only failed to provide adequate relief of their pain but, also in some cases, their bunions actually grew back.

Women seem to suffer more problems with bunions then men, no doubt due to the demands of "fashionable" footwear. Narrow and pointy-toed shoes, high heels, and other "attractive" designs push the big toe into a position that makes it even harder for it to work as designed, placing more pressure at its base and magnifying the negative impact of walking on hard surfaces.

Orthotics Use

It's not unusual for new patients who come to my office to have a history of orthotic use. The vast majority of them inform me that they eventually had to stop wearing them because they proved to be too uncomfortable for their feet, or they caused aches and pains in their knees, hips, or other areas of their body. Although some people find orthotics helpful—and those with really flat feet who overpronate may in fact benefit from them—there are two main reasons why so many others cannot tolerate them.

First, when you brace a part of the body you essentially take away the job of the individual muscles, tendons, and ligaments of the area and, therefore, they weaken (already a problem for feet stuck in shoes all day, as you well know by now). This is why many osteopaths, chiropractors, and other practitioners recommend using braces or support belts—whether for the ankles, knees, or the lower back—sparingly, or only during strenuous physical activity. The problem with orthotics, which act as braces or supports for the foot, is that they're intended to be worn all the time—to keep the positioning of the foot consistent—resulting in a weaker foot.

The second reason that people often abandon their orthotics is that unless specific steps are taken to allow the body to adjust and accommodate to them (beyond just a gradual increase in wearing time), they can create a major upheaval in all areas of the body. It's not an exaggeration to say that orthotics completely change the foundation of the body, altering the position of the foot and therefore of the ankle, knee, hip, and spine. A middle-aged or older adult's body has generally adopted a fairly well-formed inflexible pattern, or mold, and will have a hard time accommodating to the new foundation.

For those patients who arrive at my office wearing new orthotics or who get them elsewhere while in my care, I find it necessary to regularly treat them with hands-on work and instruct them to do the range-of-motion exercises for the lower body. This combination relaxes their mold and creates more "space" within the body, giving them a better chance to tolerate the stress that a changing pattern creates.

Heel Lifts

While heel lifts are less commonly prescribed than orthotics, they're also frequently abandoned by people who have worn them for similar reasons—difficulty getting used to them due to new aches and pains in the body. Since heel lifts are used on only one side, the asymmetric change they create can be even more difficult for the body to adapt to than the foundational changes created by orthotics. And although there may be some people that benefit from heel lifts (people with a history of a childhood growth-plate fracture for instance, or adults with recent joint replacement surgery), Mother Nature is very exacting and rarely creates legs of significantly different lengths. Most diagnosed leg-length discrepancies are more a function of misalignment and tension in the pelvis and joints, and should not be treated with heel lifts.

Shoe Inserts

While challenges exist with orthotic and heel-lift use, inexpensive gel or foam over-the-counter shoe inserts are generally well-tolerated by everyone. Along with well-made shoes, these are your best defense against the impact of walking on all of the hard surfaces that cover the modern world, while still allowing the muscles, ligaments, tendons, and bones of the feet to stay somewhat active and involved in the process of walking.

Treating the Cause

Rather than focus solely on the end results of the molding process as it affects the lower body (the labral tears, bursitis, and tendinitis of the hip; the meniscal tears of the knee; and the plantar fasciitis and bunions of the feet), we need to aim our treatment approach at the source—the misalignment and tension. Otherwise, there's little chance of a permanent cure and a high probability of chronic pain and future recurrences.

PHYSICALLY "BROKE"

Imagine showing up at an appointment with your financial advisor and being told that the reason you're broke is that you have no money in your bank account. While that observation may be true, it doesn't tell you anything about the cause of your being broke, nor does it offer you a solution to your problem. Being the nice individual that she is, and one who doesn't want to see you in financial pain, your advisor says she'd like to put $100 into your bank account as a remedy. Sooner or later, though, the money is spent and you're right back where you started—broke and in financial pain.

Similarly, you might hear from your doctor that you have hip or knee pain because you have bursitis or tendinitis. Your doctor is another nice individual who doesn't want to see you in pain, and so she offers to give you a steroid injection or a prescription for anti-inflammatory or pain-relieving pills. But once those medications wear off, you're right back where you started. It would be a lot more useful to address the problem by looking at the habits that are causing the misalignment and friction in the body that lead to bursitis and tendinitis—or the bleeding of the bank account—as a way to permanently solve it.

It's important to acknowledge that there are cases where severe damage within the joint has occurred—joint space narrowing to the point of bone-on-bone contact is an example—which can cause pain and dysfunction. While these cases may require surgical intervention in order to return to pain-free functioning, they're a lot rarer than most people realize.

The Proof, As They Say

If in fact the source of many people's hip and knee pain is not in those X-ray and MRI findings but instead in their gripped and tight joints and other areas, then conservative treatment approaches should prove effective. Well, the proof, as they say, is in the pudding.

The Department of Orthopedic Surgery at the Washington University School of Medicine recruited 52 outpatient orthopedic clinic patients with pre-arthritic intra-articular hip disorders—including labral tears, developmental hip dysplasia, and femoroacetabular impingement. The patients in the study completed a three-month course of conservative care for their hip complaints. One year later, 44% of the patients who had the conservative care had improved significantly, prompting the authors to conclude, "These data suggest that a trial of conservative management...should be considered before engaging in surgical intervention."[29]

The Department of Physiotherapy at Rehabtjänst, in Stockholm, Sweden, conducted a study comparing the results between two groups of knee-pain patients with documented medial meniscus tears. One group had arthroscopic partial medial meniscectomy followed by supervised exercise, and the other group was treated with supervised exercise only. At the end of the study the authors concluded that the outcome of the group that had the surgery was "not superior to supervised exercise alone in terms of reduced knee pain, improved knee function, and improved quality of life."[30]

Let's Get Started

It's time to start dedicating a few minutes every day to maintaining our human frame and improving the quality of our lives. As mentioned in an earlier Zone chapter, it's important that you understand that studies have not only demonstrated that exercises work, but also that *home-based* exercises are often as effective at reducing pain and improving function as those supervised by a physio-therapist.[31, 32] So while I encourage you to get the help of knowledgeable outside practitioners like physical therapists for support and guidance, you need to do the exercises at home, too. No exercise program will help you unless you follow it!

ZONE 3 PROGRAM: The Lower Body

STRETCHING		
EXERCISE	REP	DURATION
Piriformis on the Floor (both sides), page 78	1	:30 x 2
Hamstrings (both sides), page 79	1	:30 x 2
Quadriceps (both sides), page 80	1	:30 x 2
STRENGTHENING		
Gluteals, Hamstrings, & Quadriceps, page 81	1	:30
RANGE-OF-MOTION		
Knee Circles (two directions), page 84	1	:15 x 2
Total time of daily workout		4:00

The key to both curing and preventing lower body pain and problems is to do some targeted exercises to release the outward (or the less-common inward) rotational pull of the lower extremity. The stretching exercises will *loosen* short and tight rotator muscles, and the strengthening exercises will *strengthen* the thigh and butt muscles. The range-of-motion exercises then help to *lubricate* and *release tension* in the joints. Taken together, these exercises improve the positioning of the legs, ease the strain on and stabilize the joints, and allow for self-repair and pain relief.

NOTE: Make sure you've read Chapter Two (page 14) for important general information about the use of these exercises.

Hold all stretches a minimum of 30 seconds and do each at least once.

Piriformis Stretch on the Floor

The piriformis stretch shown below is offered as an alternative to the seated one recommended on page 55. Rather than sitting in a chair, this version is performed on the floor. Many people find the seated version easier, but both are equally effective. Choose the one that's more convenient.

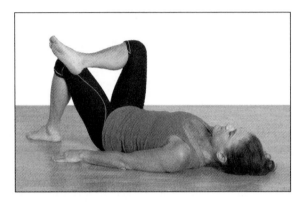

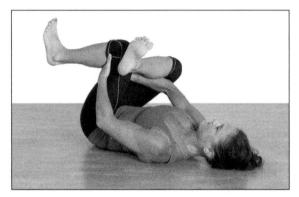

1. Lying on your back with your knees bent and feet flat on the floor, bring your right ankle to rest on top of your left thigh, just above the knee.

2. Gently hinge at the waist, reaching for your left thigh as you bring your legs up toward your trunk, until you feel a stretch in your thigh/butt area. Make sure to keep your head on the floor and your neck straight and relaxed (use a pillow under your head if necessary).

Hamstring Stretch

Though we haven't talked specifically about the hamstrings (back of the thigh) and quadriceps muscles (front of the thigh), they're very important players in the action of the lower limbs. Pain anywhere in the pelvic, hip, or butt area can arise from tight hamstrings, which tilt the pelvis backward. This simple stretch will loosen the muscles and improve the position of the pelvis.

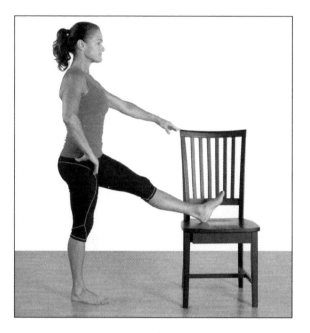

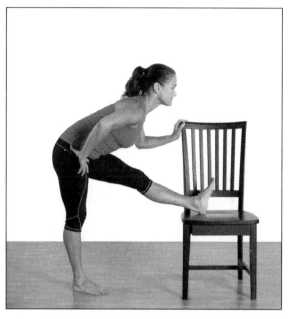

1. Stand with your right leg straight out in front of you, heel resting on a chair seat, ottoman, or similar object.

2. Bend forward at the hip joint without slouching or rounding your back.

You should feel a gentle stretch in the back of your right thigh.

Repeat on the other side.

Quadriceps Stretch

Pain in the front of the hip is often the result of tight and overworked quadriceps muscles that have been forced, due to weak and tight psoas muscles, to take over primary responsibility for the function of walking. Knee pain is also a common result of weak and tight quadriceps.

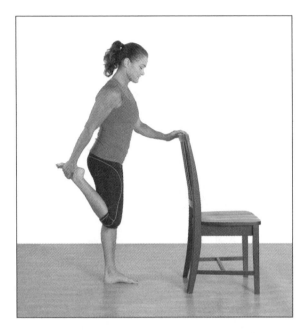

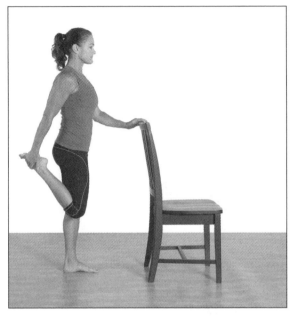

1. Standing with your left hand holding the back of a chair or other object for balance, bend your right knee and grab the ankle behind you with your right hand. Your right knee should be pointing down toward the floor.

2. While holding the ankle in place, stand nice and tall, pushing your pelvis slightly forward (imagine the right front pocket of your pants being thrust forward).

You should feel a gentle stretch in the front of the right thigh.

Repeat on the other side.

MODIFICATION: If you can't reach your ankle, loop a belt around it and grab that.

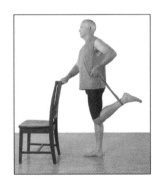

Hold or maintain all strengthening exercises a minimum of 30 seconds and do each at least once.

Gluteals, Hamstrings, & Quadriceps

The muscles of the lower body that have the most to gain from strengthening are the butt (gluteals) and thigh (hamstrings and quadriceps) muscles. These very important and powerful muscles suffer from too much sitting and general inactivity and are responsible for a lot of the pain and problems of the hips and knees (as well as the inability to easily arise from a sitting position as we get older). Fortunately, the one strengthening exercise below strengthens the gluteals, quadriceps, and hamstring muscles all at the same time.

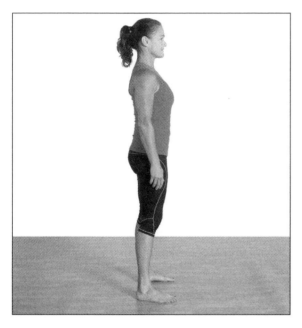

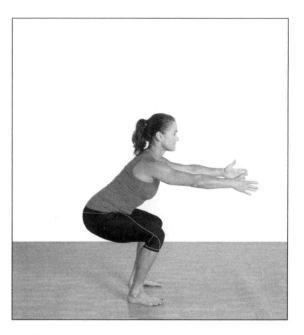

1. From a standing position, move your feet so that they're slightly wider than shoulder width with toes pointing just slightly toward the sides.

2. Slowly bend your knees and hips, lowering your body as if you were going to sit down. Keep your upper body and lower back straight—without stooping or leaning forward—and extend your arms out in front of you for balance. To avoid undue strain on your knees, keep your weight on your heels as you go into the squat, and don't let your knees move forward past the level of your toes. Also, imagine you're standing on a towel and you're spreading it wider with your feet as you squat down. This will keep your knees from buckling inward. If possible, squat down far enough so that your thighs become parallel to the ground. Don't be discouraged if you need to work up to this. It's hard! (See note below.)

Hold this position for 3 seconds and then *slowly* begin to straighten your legs until you're standing upright again.

Repeat 10 to 12 times, once a day, 3 times a week, with a day or two of rest in between sessions.

NOTE: Some people can't squat low enough to get their thighs parallel to the ground (which is necessary in order to strengthen the gluteal muscles) due to pain in the knees or the inability to get back up. If that's true for you, do the squats while dropping as low as you comfortably can to strengthen the thigh muscles, and add the alternate version exercise below to strengthen the gluteal muscles.

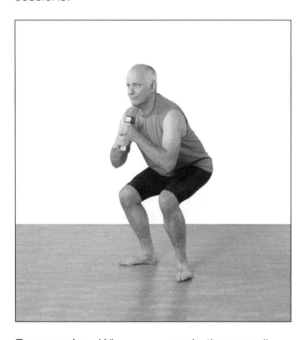

Progression: When you can do these easily, hold a medicine ball or other weight in your arms to make it more challenging.

ALTERNATE VERSION: While not as complete a lower-body strengthening exercise, if squatting proves too difficult due to balance, weakness, or joint pain problems, try this exercise:

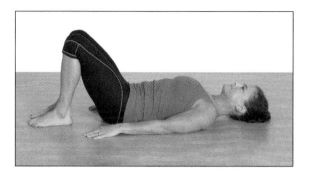

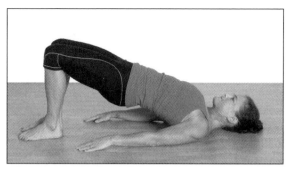

1. Lie on your back on the floor, knees bent and feet flat on the ground.

2. Press your weight into your heels and lift your pelvis up off the floor, creating a straight line from your trunk to your knees. Keep your head and neck relaxed as you tighten your glutes.

Hold for 3 seconds, then slowly lower your pelvis back down to the floor.

Repeat 10 to 12 times, once a day, 3 times a week, with a day or two of rest in between sessions.

Perform range-of-motion maneuvers a minimum of 15 seconds and do each at least once.

Knee Circles

Although referred to as knee circles, this exercise is a simple but effective technique to loosen the joints of the knees, ankles, and feet. Many of my older patients' ankles and feet have become stiff, compromising the ability of the feet to position themselves properly when walking, and inhibiting their ability to perform the very important job of shock absorption. Tension in these joints not only leads to chronic local pain and problems, but also compromises the hips, pelvis, and lower back since the legs and feet are the foundation that the rest of the body rests upon.

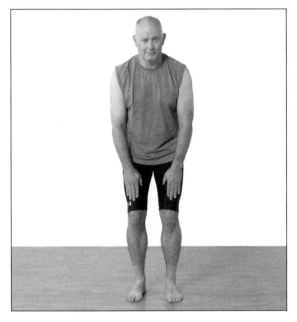
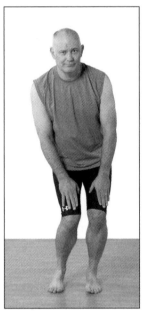
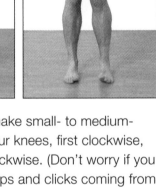

1. From a standing position, feet a couple of inches apart, bend slightly at the hips and knees and place your hands on your thighs just above your knees. (Remember, whenever you bend at the hips, you should be aware of your butt sticking out behind you and your lower back being straight.)

2. Slowly begin to make small- to medium-sized circles with your knees, first clockwise, and then counterclockwise. (Don't worry if you hear some minor pops and clicks coming from your joints as you do the exercise.)

Do 10 to 15 circles in each direction.

CHAPTER SIX
The Ten-Minute-a-Day Program

Those who do not find time for exercise will have to find time for illness.

—Edward Stanley

Beginning with Chapter Seven, the rest of this book is dedicated to the two other tools and important recommendations for self-treatment to end everyday pain. As you'll discover, those tools and suggestions don't take a specific amount of time but instead are things that can—and should—be incorporated into your daily routine as needed. Before moving on, however, let's take a moment to summarize the individual zone approach and then put it all together into the ten-minute-a-day program of stretching, strengthening, and movement.

As previously mentioned, the purpose of focusing on individual zones is to target the exercises to the specific region that you're having pain and problems in. It utilizes one of the most powerful tools to break the grip of misalignment and tension in a minimal amount of time. It also introduces you to the habit of spending a few minutes every day working on your own body—if you aren't doing so already—and starts you on the road to recovery and improved health.

If you're not currently in pain, however, or are motivated to do the exercises for more than one zone, I encourage you to get into the habit of doing the whole ten-minute-a-day program right from the start. In addition to treating any specific areas you may be troubled by, doing all of the exercises is essential to maintain the health of the body and prevent new problems from arising.

Regardless of which way you begin, the ultimate goal is to do the full program every day. The following page lists all of the exercises—consolidated from the three individual zones for easy reference—targeted to break the grip and end everyday pain.

STRETCHING		
EXERCISE	REP	DURATION
Shoulder & Chest, page 32	1	:30
Upper Back, Shoulder, & Neck, page 34	1	:30
Neck, page 35	1	:30
Psoas, page 53	1	:30
Piriformis (both sides), page 55 or page 78	1	:30 x 2
Gluteals (both sides), page 56	1	:30 x 2
Hamstrings (both sides), page 79	1	:30 x 2
Quadriceps (both sides), page 80	1	:30 x 2
STRENGTHENING		
Rhomboids, page 37	1	:30
Spinal Extensors, page 57	1	:30
Gluteals, Hamstrings, & Quadriceps, page 81	1	:30
RANGE-OF-MOTION		
Shoulder Rolls, page 38	1	:30
Flexion/Extension, page 59	1	:30
Side Bending, page 60	1	:30
Rotation, page 61	1	:30
Knee Circles (two directions), page 84	1	:15 x 2
Total time of daily workout		10:00

CHAPTER SEVEN

The Crowbar: Habit Modification

First we form habits, then they form us. Conquer your bad habits or they will conquer you.

—Rob Gilbert

By now you're acquainted with the stretches, strengthening, and range-of-motion exercises because you've read the chapter(s) for whichever zone(s) you're having problems with. While movement is incredibly powerful—I dubbed it "The Hammer," remember?—it has been my experience that people are best able to break the grip and end everyday pain when they incorporate all of the tools laid out in this book. While the percentage of time devoted to each can vary, some combination of targeted movement, habit modification, and the expertise of an outside practitioner generally gets the job done faster, more thoroughly, and with less effort. Now let's turn our attention to habit modification.

Change Some Habits, Change Your Life

Through the years I've identified some very common habits engaged in by my patients that over time result in misalignment and tension. Modifying those habits, breaking their grip, is a subtle but effective tool. I've dubbed this tool "The Crowbar" because, as with a crowbar, just a little effort on one end can have a surprisingly effective leveraging action at the other end.

Of all the habits I've identified, one of the most common and most damaging is the general tendency for adults to move less frequently and in more repetitive ways. When we were younger, we played at the park on the jungle gym, the swings, and the slide; we climbed trees, played hopscotch, and participated in sports, using our bodies in all sorts of varied ways. Different activities called upon different muscles used in different combinations. As adults, however, we vastly restrict our movements through such things as specialized and repetitive jobs, sitting and working at desks, commuting in cars and trains, using remote controls, drive-in windows, and automatic garage-door openers.

In addition to this general trend of moving less, we've also adopted habits that over time can mold our bodies and create problems, such as always sleeping on one's side, using pillows that are the wrong size, and reading or watching television while lying down. Whenever I interview a new patient with chronic aches and pains, I always include questions about these and other habits.

Posture

If you're like most people, you really don't want to talk about your posture, that nagging thing we all know we should improve but rarely do. Well, I think I can make improving your posture easy for you, but before we get into that, let me just say that, yes, posture is important. *Correct posture is our main defense against the effects of gravity.* If you doubt the power of gravity, think about all of those picturesque stone walls that line the fields and the woods in many parts of the country. As heavy and as solid as they may be, if stone walls are not built upright and true, gravity will eventually wear them down. A properly aligned and built stone wall, on the other hand, will resist the forces bearing on it and remain upright and sturdy.

The same is true for the human body. The human neck, for example, was designed to support the weight of the head above it. Move the head just one inch forward, however (a common postural event for middle-aged and older people), and the weight the neck has to support essentially doubles. This sets the stage for a whole host of problems (the wall begins to fall!), not the least of which is chronic neck pain. Fortunately, posture is a learned behavior and therefore can be improved upon at any time.

Regardless of which strategies for postural improvement you employ (and I'll show you targeted ones in a minute that have worked for many of my patients), just remember that no method will be very successful unless you also do some stretches and range-of-motion exercises. The reason for this is that whenever you forget to pay attention to your posture—which initially, at least, will be almost all the time—the tension in your body will pull you right back into the old mold. Not only will these exercises help you avoid that problem, but they can also lessen the pain that almost inevitably comes when you start to engage muscles and other structures that may have been ignored for a long time. If you've ever tried something as simple as trying to improve your posture by sitting more upright at your desk instead of slouching, you know that this can cause temporary discomfort or even pain in your back. What you're doing is asking muscles and other structures that have long been unemployed to get back to work. Initially, these muscles might not appreciate the opportunity to get back on the job, but that doesn't mean that improving your posture isn't better and more desirable in the long run. Stretching and range-of-motion exercises will get you through this painful part more quickly, or even eliminate it altogether.

Based on my patients' experiences, I can say with certainty that it's much easier and therefore more effective to target strategies for postural improvement on just one or two key areas in each zone. Wherever your pain is, feel free initially to focus your efforts on changes in that zone. Eventually, try to incorporate the targeted postural strategies for all three zones. I've kept the strategies short and to the point to make the whole process easy.

Targeted Postural Strategies for the Upper Body

The two key areas of the upper body to focus on when you're starting to address your posture are the head and shoulders. As previously discussed, the most common problem with the head position of my older patients is that it's not in proper alignment with the trunk, but is jutting forward in front of it. A more properly situated head, on the other hand, requires very little work from the neck and back muscles and actually helps to elongate the cervical spine, counteracting the downward pressure of gravity and keeping the discs less compressed and healthier.

Similarly, the most common postural problem with the shoulders is that they round forward over time. This pulls the shoulder blades away from the spine, narrows the subacromial space, and creates problems for the upper back and neck muscles (*rhomboids, trapezius, and levator scapulae*), the rotator cuff tendons, and the bursae of the shoulders.

Here are some tips to help you improve the posture of the upper body by improving the position of the head and shoulders:

1. If you use a desktop computer, position the monitor in such a way that you have to look slightly down at it, allowing the back of the neck to stay elongated (see figure 6.1 on page 90).

2. When reading at a desk or table, place the reading material on a book stand—or put a coffee mug (or similarly sized object) on the desk, under the top part of the book—rather than lay it flat on the surface. The goal is to angle the book about 30 degrees up from flat on the desk. Elevating the material in this way places your head in a better position—not looking down too much—creating less strain on the neck and upper back muscles.

3. If you're sitting at a table or desk using a keypad or a mouse, pull the chair close enough so that you don't have to lean forward—a position that encourages rounding of the shoulders.

4. When sitting in a chair, try to rest your elbows on the arms of the chair or other such surface, or to keep your hands resting on the tops of your upper thighs. Avoid resting them in your lap between your legs, which pulls your shoulders forward.

5. When driving, sit as close to the wheel as you can comfortably (while allowing room for the airbag should it deploy) so that your arms aren't reaching too far forward. The seat back should be as upright as possible to allow the head and neck to sit atop the trunk without craning forward.

Postural Cue for the Upper Body

To help keep the head positioned properly, imagine a line that starts at your ear and extends through your eyes, pointing slightly down (figure 6-1). This is a slight tilting action, not a nodding forward of the whole head. Your chin should also feel like it's also pointing down a little (the image of a tennis ball held under your chin—in the fold of the neck—may help) so that the back of the neck is being elongated.

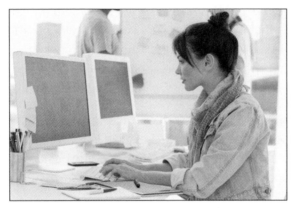

Figure 6-1

Targeted Postural Strategies for the Lower Back

The most common postural problems of the lower back arise when the normal curve of the lumbar spine is reduced. The health of the discs between the vertebrae, and of the muscles and soft tissues surrounding the spine, rely on the proper position of the lumbar curve. Sitting incorrectly and lifting objects improperly are two of the leading insults to the lumbar spine, resulting in recurrent lower back pain and problems.

The Proper Way to Sit

There's a growing body of evidence that suggests that the traditional way of sitting in a chair—with the trunk upright and the thighs perpendicular (at a 90-degree angle to the trunk) (figure 6-2a)—may not be the best position for your lower back. Some studies suggest that this position stresses the lumbar spine, misaligning and placing strain on the discs and associated muscles and tendons. Perhaps this explains why so many people find that their lower backs get stiff and achy after sitting in a chair or car seat for any length of time.

In contrast, sitting with a wider angle between the trunk and thigh (one that approximates 135 degrees, according to one study) was shown to be a more relaxed position and puts less stress on the lower back region. This probably explains why people like to lean back when sitting in a chair or on the couch (figure 6-2b). While leaning back—or reclining—increases the angle between the thighs and trunk and relieves lower back pressure, unfortunately, it also tends to round the upper back (slouching) and forces the head and neck to crane forward when reading or watching television.

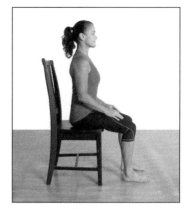

Figure 6-2a

Given our current seating options, the least stressful position for the lower back—while also allowing for good upright upper body posture—might be achieved by sitting on a tilted-forward chair seat, if that's an option, or by sitting on a wedge-shaped cushion. For years, I've found myself approximating this position by sitting on the front edge of my desk chair, with my thighs angled down toward the floor, and my legs folded underneath me resting on the base of the chair.

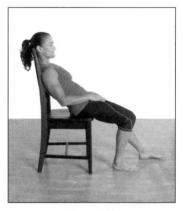

Figure 6-2b

Regardless of which method you choose—tilted seat, wedge-shaped cushion, or perched on the front edge of the seat (figure 6-2c) (don't worry about the exact angle, 135 degrees is probably not a realistic sitting position anyway)—be sure to make this adjustment gradually. Your body has adapted to the way you sit currently and changing it will require new muscles to get active (usually creating some mid-back soreness). Take frequent breaks and do your targeted movement exercises to ease the transition.

The Proper Way to Lift

People who suffer from lower back pain can frequently trace the origin of their pain to lifting something. Many of them are surprised at just how little weight it actually took to set their back off. What they don't realize is that the *way* you lift is just as important as *how much weight* you lift, if not more so. The key is to avoid bending at the back—rounding it and hunching over—as so many people do. Rounding over in this way, even without picking up anything heavy, puts tremendous pressure on the muscles and discs of the lower

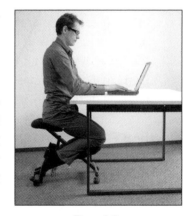

Figure 6-2c

back; the weight of the forward-bending upper body combined with the forces of gravity is already a burden to a rounded spine before the additional weight of the object to be lifted is added.

To avoid injuring yourself while lifting, follow these easy rules:

1. Perhaps the most important rule of lifting is that whenever you bend over, whether to pick something up, tie your shoes, or pull a weed, you need to *hinge at the hip joints*, keeping the lower back curve intact. This will require you to stick your butt way out behind you, almost as if to arch your back just slightly (figure 6-3a). Most people bend from their lower backs, going against the normal curvature and thereby putting a lot of pressure on the discs between the vertebrae and on the supporting muscles and other soft tissues (figure 6-3b). If you think of keeping your back straight while bending over, this will help you not to round.

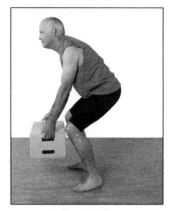

Figure 6-3a

2. When lifting an object, bend your knees and use your powerful thigh and butt muscles to do the heavy work. Simply focusing your attention on those muscles will ease the burden on your lower back.

3. Keep the objects that you're lifting close to your body; try to keep a bend in your elbows so that you don't have your arms fully outstretched when lifting.

4. When maneuvering a heavy object, avoid making more than one movement at a time, such as turning and bending simultaneously. Rather than twisting to put something down in one fluid movement (like lifting a grocery bag out of the cart

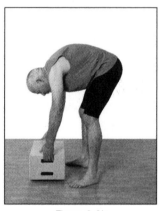

Figure 6-3b

and then turning your upper body 90 degrees while leaning forward to place the bag into the trunk of your car), turn your whole body first, then stop and then bend to put it down. Combinations of movements create extra demand on the spine and soft tissues and can result in disc injuries and muscle spasms.

Postural Cue for the Lower Back

Whether you're sitting in a chair, lifting a bag of pet food from the trunk, or even just leaning over a sink brushing your teeth or washing dishes, assume a posture that makes you aware of your butt out behind you with your lower back gently and naturally arched. You should feel that you're hinging your forward-bending movements at the hip joints—not at the lumbar spine itself. While sticking your butt out behind you will probably feel silly or seem like an exaggerated position at first, before long you may appreciate how much better it makes your lower back feel. Take a look at pictures of adults who work bending over—people who pick crops or lay bricks for a living—and you will see how they push their butts out, thereby maintaining the normal curve of the lower back. Consciously or unconsciously, they're protecting their lower backs (figure 6-4).

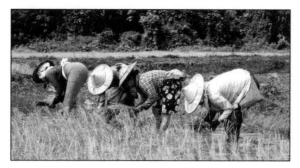

Figure 6-4

Targeted Postural Strategies for the Lower Body

The postural problems of the lower body typically revolve around the positioning of the lower limbs, most commonly where the legs and feet point more toward the sides than straight ahead. This means that rather than hinging straight back and forth as designed, following a mostly forward-facing foot, the joints of the misaligned lower extremities are forced to add a rotational movement, creating problems for the feet, knees, and hips. Consequently, it's important to be aware of the position of the legs not only when standing and walking, but also when sitting and lying down.

Here are some tips for improving the posture of the lower body by correcting the position of the lower extremities:

1. Don't cross your legs when you sit. Keep your feet flat on the floor with toes pointing mostly straight ahead to prevent the hips from externally rotating.

2. Similarly, when you lie down on your back, don't cross your legs at your ankles. Children rarely do this, but adults frequently do because it's a more comfortable position for the misaligned legs of adulthood.

3. When walking, try to keep the feet pointing roughly straight ahead instead of inward or diagonally out toward the sides. Although this orientation may feel strange at first, after a few weeks it will feel more natural and you won't have to think so hard about it.

Postural Cue for the Lower Body

This one is simple: When you walk, try to take longer strides or, as I sometimes say, walk with a purpose. We have a tendency to meander, or shuffle along, taking short strides when we walk. This keeps the feet pointing more toward the sides. When you take a nice long step, the foot must point more forward when it finally hits the ground.

Check In with Yourself

Get into the habit of checking in with yourself periodically throughout the day about your posture and positioning. The more you catch yourself compromising your positioning and then correcting it—head perched high with the back of the neck elongated, lower back curve maintained, legs and feet pointing mostly straight ahead—the more aware you'll become, and the better off you'll be.

Take Breaks from Sitting

One very common problem of life in the world today is that we frequently spend long hours engaged in physically limiting activities, which can be especially challenging to the body if they require us to sit while doing them. Many of my lower back, hip, and knee pain patients discover that their joints begin to ache during prolonged sitting. This tells me that static positions are not good for the body—a body that's designed to move—and that if we get stuck in one position for too long—even one that's relatively correct—our muscles and other structures get tight and tense.

It's extremely important to make a habit of taking movement breaks during periods of prolonged inactivity. Not only does sitting mold the body, but it also seems to actually be dangerous in itself. Recent evidence suggests that too much sitting may be an independent risk factor for heart disease and cancer! So whether you're doing office work at a desk (you may want to consider a standing desk), using a computer at home, or sitting on the couch knitting or watching television, you need to get up every 20 minutes or so and move around. Yes, every 20 minutes. (If you're driving in the car, try to get out and move around once an hour.) Get up, stand tall, and, while you're standing there, spend a minute or two doing some of the range-of-motion exercises listed for the Three Zones of the body. The mere act of standing and stretching will reset the clock that marks the time you've spent sitting and will help you avoid postural strain.

Sleeping Positions

Considering that we spend almost a third of our lives in bed, it should come as no surprise that our sleep habits affect the body profoundly and are crucial to consider in relationship to our structural health. Following just a few basic guidelines can be of tremendous support in leading a pain-free life.

As I've discovered through my own patient population, there appears to be a correlation between side sleepers and shoulder and hip problems. The likely problem for the shoulders is that when you sleep on your side, your arms are not only stationed in front of your body, rounding the shoulders, but also the pressure from the mattress forces the bottom shoulder even further forward. The end result is more shoulder impingement and further strengthening of the mold.

As for the hips, pressure on the hip joint from sleeping on the side may over time compress the ball-and-socket joint, creating problems. In addition, the slightly drawn-up leg position that often accompanies side sleeping serves to further shorten the muscles of the lower back and the hips.

Sleeping on your stomach or back, in contrast, doesn't place any pressure directly on the shoulder or hip joints and doesn't further solidify the common mold. Though stomach sleeping is often advised against because of the potential stress it can create on the spine, it's probably okay unless you suffer from lower back or neck stiffness or pain. If you sleep on your back, try not to use a pillow under your knees unless you're suffering from lower back pain. Allowing the hip flexor muscles of the lower back to lengthen at night—which happens when your legs are extended straight out while sleeping—is beneficial to those muscles.

Another option that many people find helpful, and one I typically recommend as an alternative to side sleeping, is to sleep at something of a 45-degree angle using a couple of pillows—or one body pillow—either behind your back or in front of your chest to keep you positioned. Compared to side sleeping, sleeping at an angle takes most of the pressure off the shoulders and hips, does less to reinforce the mold, and is usually well tolerated by those needing to change from their current position because of pain.

Pillow Heights

Without even knowing it, many people are in the habit of sleeping with a pillow that isn't the correct thickness, leading to molding and chronic pain in the neck, shoulders, upper back, and head. The most important consideration when it comes to pillow thickness is choosing one that puts the head and neck in the correct relationship to the trunk when you sleep. In general, back and front sleepers should use a very thin pillow as the head is already naturally aligned in those positions, and side sleepers should use a thicker one that's high enough to fill in the space between the head and the shoulder on the mattress (figure 6-5).

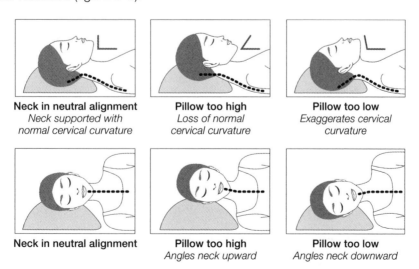

Figure 6-5. Proper pillow heights for all sleeping positions

These guidelines break down, however, in the case of older adults whose posture has forced their heads forward and who sleep on their backs. As we learned in Chapter Three, older adults with this kind of forward molding require increased pillow height or else the head will be tilted back uncomfortably, putting strain on the neck (hyperextending it). If you fall into this category, choose a pillow height that's currently comfortable for you. At the same time, make it a goal to slowly transition to a thinner pillow, doing the stretches, range-of-motion exercises, and postural cues for Zone 1 daily in order to help you with the transition. Some good hands-on treatment will also support you in achieving this goal.

Reading & Watching Television while Lying Down

Reading and watching television while lying in bed or on the couch, head propped-up on pillows, are such regular and frequent habits for so many people that they may do more to mold and grip the adult body than any other activities, except perhaps sitting in a slouched position. Although these activities might be comfortable (in the short term) and enjoyable, they put a lot of strain on

the upper body. Rather than lying down, try to sit up in a chair (with a wedge-shaped cushion) next to the bed or couch, maintaining your lower back curve, and keeping your head aligned with your trunk. And remember to take frequent breaks!

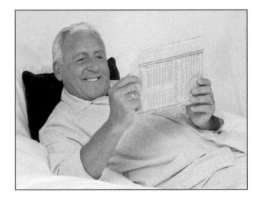

That being said, patients who have a hard time giving up this very popular but compromising habit may not have to forego that pleasure entirely if they increase the time spent on targeted movement and outside treatment. Although identifying and then modifying some of your bad postural habits is an important tool for pain-free living, I wouldn't dream of demanding that you give up all of them! If you devote more time to other strategies—do the targeted movement exercises regularly and get your body treated—you may well be able to continue these challenging activities without suffering the consequences.

Avoid the "Weekend Warrior" Syndrome

Try to avoid the habit of sitting all week with little or no physical activity only to ramp up the physical exertion level on weekends. Weekend warriors, as they're sometimes referred to, are plentiful in our pressed-for-time world, and they frequently show up in offices like mine on Monday mornings with serious aches and pains. Once again, an ounce of prevention is worth a pound of cure.

As I'm sure you understand by now, the spine, muscles, and joints of the body become misaligned, tight, and weak when you're perched at a desk, in a car, or on the couch all week long. When the weekend comes around and the body is asked to engage full force in physical activities like swinging a tennis racquet or a golf club, swimming, running, biking, or even gardening, it frequently rebels. Muscles go into spasm, tendons tear, bursa get irritated and inflamed, and nerves get pinched.

Don't get me wrong. It's not that I prefer that you stay sedentary on the weekends, it's that I'd like you to be more active during the week as well. A little dedicated effort Monday through Friday is all it takes to keep your body fit and prepared for more activity on the weekends, if that's what you desire. It doesn't take a lot, I promise. Doing daily stretches and range-of-motion exercises will not only ease the tension in your body and break the grip that molding has created, it will have the added benefit of preparing your musculoskeletal system for weekend activities and challenges. Otherwise, in all likelihood, I'll see you in my office on Monday morning!

Big Dividends

It doesn't take a lot of effort to move the body a little bit more, adjust reading and television-watching positions, or take short breaks during long drives or when doing desk work. I'm quite sure that if you pay attention to your own daily routines you'll find many more instances where you're compromising the body and advancing your mold. Once you become aware of them, the process of modifying your bad habits becomes relatively easy yet pays big dividends.

CHAPTER EIGHT

The Carpenter: Outside Practitioners

When you have adjusted the physical to its normal demands,
Nature universally supplies the remainder.

—A. T. Still

An outside practitioner is someone outside of the modern medical community who sees and treats you as a whole and not just a lot of unrelated parts. In that respect, he or she is *(w)holistic*. An outside practitioner is also interested in finding the cause of pain and disease as opposed to being content just treating the symptoms (this is not to say that all medical doctors are content to just treat symptoms). For the purposes of this book, my focus is on outside practitioners whose main area of interest is the human frame and who utilize a hands-on approach in the treatment of it.

By now you're familiar with the targeted-movement and habit-modification tools—the Hammer and the Crowbar. This final tool incorporates the skills of an outside practitioner, the person I call the "Carpenter." As a part-time do-it-yourselfer, I can attest to the fact that if a project is complicated—or you really want it done right—sometimes you need to call in an expert. It's my personal belief that we can all benefit from a little expert help in this world, whether it's for the repair of a home, a car, or our physical bodies. There's no point in trying to build walls that are level and square, for instance, if your understanding of the process is incomplete and you don't have the right tools. When that's the case, not only will you be frustrating yourself and possibly damaging or wasting supplies, but you'll also be delaying the moment when you have the result you want.

The role of the outside practitioner, the individual who's had specialty training, is both to advance your progress in ways that would be difficult—if not impossible—for you to do yourself, and to fine-tune that progress as a carpenter does for a building project. If you've spent years in chronic pain, you may get the quickest relief by initially devoting the largest percentage of time and effort to being treated by a skilled outside practitioner. They have many tools at their disposal, and their ability to realign the body and reduce damage-causing tension can eliminate pain and set the stage for self-repair.

As you begin to feel improvements, you can often maintain your results even as you reduce the number of visits to the practitioner—as long as you increase the time spent doing the targeted-movement exercises and incorporate a few of the habit changes outlined in this book.

No matter which type of outside practitioner you choose, remember that although the practitioner plays an important and necessary role in your healing and health maintenance, most of what needs to be done to care for your body can and must be done by *you* on a daily basis.

Consider the following when you're looking for an outside practitioner and starting treatment:

1. It's always a good idea to ask people you know for recommendations based on their own experience. There's nothing like a referral from a trusted source.

2. Don't be afraid to call practitioners and ask questions. They should be able to give you clear and specific information about the type of treatment they employ, the anticipated duration of the treatment program, the results you can expect, and the cost.

3. My patients often ask me if it's okay to be treated by multiple outside practitioners at one time in a sort of shotgun approach. Though this may get good results for you, it can make it more difficult to identify where the results are coming from. Additionally, it is possible to be overtreated (see below).

4. The body needs rest between treatments to recover and to incorporate the changes that are being instituted. Avoid overtreatment, or multiple treatments in a short period of time by one or more practitioners.

5. In general, by the time most people seek help, their bodies have been gripped and molded over many years. Therefore, even with the assistance of a skilled outside practitioner, it may take some time to break the grip and begin to feel changes. Monitor your progress and be patient.

6. It isn't always easy to know if treatments are working in the short term, especially because the pain sometimes gets worse or changes its nature or location before it gets better. (This can be a treatment reaction, discussed more at the end of this chapter.) Let your intuition be your guide. If you have a sense that the practitioner is skillful and feel that things are changing, then stay with it. If the practitioner doesn't seem to be taking your concerns seriously enough, or the pain seems intuitively wrong, then it's probably a good idea to look for someone else.

In this chapter, I'll focus on the most commonly available treatment modalities. Many more modalities exist, of course, and just because I don't include something here doesn't mean that it's not worthwhile. For a variety of reasons, different people respond to different treatment modalities differently. Said another way, you'll respond to some approaches and practitioners better than to others. It bears repeating that one of the best ways to find great practitioners is to ask friends for referrals. Along with talking to friends and doctors, do some online research to find out what's available in your area.

ABOUT OSTEOPATHY

Osteopathy is an American-born medical approach pioneered in the late 19th century by a frontier physician, surgeon, Civil War officer, and statesman named Andrew Taylor Still, MD, DO (1828–1917). Dr. Still's disdain of the orthodox medical practices of his day stemmed from his firsthand experience of their ineffectiveness (he suffered the tragic loss of three of his children to meningitis) as well as their clear potential for harm (many medical remedies of the day were highly toxic and addictive). Being a man of great intelligence and compassion, he questioned the approach of traditional medicine and sought an alternative and more effective system of healing. Dr. Still's intense study of human anatomy and physiology, along with his belief in the unity of body, mind, and spirit, and the "power of Nature to cure" were the seeds of what eventually grew into the science he called osteopathy.

Dr. Still did not claim to have invented osteopathy but merely to have discovered it—a truth "as old as the cranium itself." He believed that the human body contained within it all the necessary mechanisms for its own defense and repair in the event of a traumatic, toxic, or infectious insult, and that although the tendency in the patient's body was always to get well, an insult to the body could impair its ability to function and exert an abnormal influence on the patient as a whole. His approach to healing, therefore, centered on the use of gentle hands-on techniques to remove tension and misalignment from the human frame, freeing the forces within the patient to engage in the natural healing process. Dr. Still's philosophy and principles, espoused over 100 years ago yet still valid today, created the foundation of an art and science of medicine with a truly holistic approach.

Osteopathic Manipulation

Osteopathic manipulation is practiced by doctors of osteopathy (DOs) who, like MDs, attend four years of medical school followed by specialty residency training. With their medical background and experience, osteopathic physicians are qualified to, and do, practice all branches of medicine, including surgery, but today only a handful still diagnose and treat musculoskeletal conditions using a hands-on approach. That approach, called osteopathic manipulation, is something of a lost art, and those that still practice it are hard to find. If you can find an osteopath who does manipulation, he or she will most likely employ several methods to treat the pain and problems of the body. These include gentle techniques to treat the bones and soft tissues such as balanced ligamentous tension, myofascial release, muscle energy, counter-strain, and cranial osteopathy.

Over the years, variations on many of these osteopathic techniques have been adopted and adapted by other body workers and therapists. Counter-strain and myofascial release, for example, are commonly employed by physical therapists, and an altered version of cranial osteopathy, called cranial-sacral therapy, is taught and practiced by massage therapists, chiropractors, and other non-physician practitioners. Though these and other techniques lose some of their effectiveness when removed from the osteopathic framework, they can still be very valuable.

Years ago osteopathic physicians who did hands-on manipulation employed the high-velocity, or "spine-cracking," type of adjustments to the spine more associated today with chiropractors. More recently, those osteopaths that specialize in hands-on work have largely gotten away from forceful adjustments and employ the gentler techniques mentioned above. My experience has taught me that the body responds much better to subtle methods, whether those methods are being used to treat the spine directly, or the tendons, ligaments, soft tissues, and fluids that surround it and influence it. Regardless of who is performing it, I don't recommend the more aggressive type of high-velocity adjustment to the spine, as I'll discuss further below.

Chiropractic Adjustments

Chiropractors understand very well the role of the spine as it relates to pain and problems of the body. Like other outside practitioners, they're interested in improving alignment and mobility through hands-on work, and some offer patients instruction in the use of stretching and exercise.

Like physicians, chiropractors are also trained in the art of diagnosis and frequently take X-rays as part of their work-up. Though this can be advantageous, as it yields more information, it makes them subject to a vulnerability we've discussed previously as it relates to medical doctors: homing in on a particular radiologic finding such as arthritis, a subluxation, or (something I hear frequently from my patients who have seen a chiropractor) a neck that isn't curved enough. Like many radiologic findings, these are often not the actual source of a patient's pain, and can cause practitioners to miss the bigger picture.

Chiropractic treatment styles differ widely. Some chiropractors are moving away from the traditional approach of high-velocity adjustment, where they move the head and neck or other body part quickly, often eliciting a cracking sound as the bones of the spine move. As someone who learned to give this type of adjustment in my early days of osteopathic medical school—and who received plenty of it, too—it's my opinion that this is to be avoided for two reasons. First, many people are reluctant to receive this kind of treatment because of its aggressive nature and so they instinctively tense up when it's about to be administered; I know many chiropractors who feel the need to distract the patient just prior to applying the technique in order to get them to relax. Personally, I try to listen to and heed inner feelings of reluctance whether I'm giving or receiving a treatment. Second, once the force from the practitioner is removed, there's little to maintain the change except repeating the force. This may, over time, damage the body and make you reliant on the process for continued results.

If you want to use a chiropractor—and there are many good ones out there—find one who treats the soft tissues as well as the bones, who favors gentle hands-on adjustments, and who treats the whole body and not just the upper neck or other region. Try to avoid any treatment style that requires aggressive manipulation and multiple visits per week. My experience has taught me that the body responds much better to being coaxed than bullied (makes sense, right?) and needs time between treatments to assimilate and incorporate the changes being made. Said another way, unmolding or degripping the human frame is a deliberate process of creating more space, a process that takes time and cannot be forced.

Therapeutic Massage

Therapeutic massage should be a staple component of everyone's healthy lifestyle toolbox. Let's be clear: I'm talking about *therapeutic* massage, not hot-stone or other spa-type massage treatments. Those kinds of body work, though enjoyable, are not designed to help break the grip of entrenched molding, and have given some the impression that massage is a treat to be reserved for special occasions. Therapeutic massage—also sometimes called deep-tissue or sports massage—on the other hand, has as its goal the treatment and prevention of pain-producing problems and shouldn't be viewed as a luxury.

The muscles take up a lot of room in our bodies and the benefits of keeping them happy are huge. Loosening and relaxing these tireless workers can help release tension, improve posture, and enhance circulation and lymphatic drainage (the body's waste disposal system). Whether helping to reduce the forward pull of the shoulders, ease the tight hip flexors and the lower back, or decrease the outward rotation of the lower limbs, therapeutic massage can help to reduce the aches, pains, and problems of the musculoskeletal system. At a minimum, I recommend a once-a-month visit for maintenance, and as frequently as once a week if you're suffering from pain in any area of the body.

Physical Therapy

Physical therapists are a very valuable asset as they can address the aches, pains, and problems of the body with a variety of useful hands-on techniques. Additionally, they can assist in the healing of inflamed or strained areas through the use of such things as hot and cold packs, ultrasound, and electrical stimulation. They can also provide education and guidance regarding posture, home stretching, strengthening, and mobility programs.

Physical therapists are becoming more and more relied upon to treat an increasing number of musculoskeletal conditions for which the modern medical physician can offer little more than a drug prescription. Fortunately, a skilled physical therapist can often offer relief through hands-on manipulation to address tension in the soft tissues and restrictions of the joints. One word of caution, however, is that some physical therapists seem to encourage premature strength training, often through the use of Thera-Bands. (Thera-Bands are stretchy lengths of rubber used for resistance exercises.) Though some studies may suggest a role for early strengthening exercises, the experience of many of my middle-aged and older patients is that doing resistance exercises too early worsens pain and keeps the problem smoldering. It has been my experience that an inflamed or strained area needs rest first and foremost, along with some gentle mobility exercises, and not more work. Later on, after the shoulder, hip, or knee has fully recovered, strengthening exercises can be added without the risk of further irritation and inflammation.

To their credit, many physical therapists are scrambling to learn more in order to handle the many varied and complex musculoskeletal problems that physicians send their way. They're a great treatment option since they're readily available—although they may require a doctor's prescription—and because of their interest in the human frame and because they use their hands to treat it. As with other modalities, however, the training and expertise of physical therapists varies widely—as well as the amount of supervision they offer you while you're learning the exercises—and care should be taken when choosing one.

Other Approaches

Other approaches to treating the musculoskeletal system with which I've seen people have success and that may be worth exploring include:

Pilates consists of controlled movements designed to improve alignment, increase flexibility, and build strength. Its benefits can go beyond the physical to include an improved sense of well-being.

Yoga has many definitions, but can be simplified as an ancient system of physical exercises (poses)—that many modern stretches are based on—the practice of which improves strength, flexibility, and spiritual well-being.

The Alexander Technique is a way of learning to move mindfully, exploring habits of movement and patterns of tension. It's a practical method that, once learned, can be applied in all situations to restore freedom of movement.

Feldenkrais is a form of body education that uses gentle movement and directed attention to increase range of motion, improve flexibility, and reestablish efficient movement.

Rolfing is a form of body work of the soft tissues designed to affect the body's posture and structure. It manipulates the myofascial system to ease strain patterns of the entire body.

Acupuncture is a form of Chinese medicine that's based on the theory that energy, called chi, flows through and around your body along pathways. When something blocks your chi, illness results. Very thin needles are then placed into your skin to unblock it, helping the chi return to an improved state of balance.

Personal trainers are fitness professionals involved in exercise prescription and instruction. They design programs to help their clients reach personal health and fitness goals. Some of my patients have found it beneficial to work with personal trainers, especially ones who have a particular interest in rehabilitation.

A WORD ABOUT SPINAL MANIPULATION

As a result of all of the various postural changes and traumas that we've been discussing so far, the spine itself—not just the muscles and soft tissues around it—frequently becomes misaligned and tight, which can lead to all sorts of bad outcomes: headaches; neck and upper back pain; lower back and hip pain; nerve compression that results in radiating pain, numbness, and weakness in the arms or legs; and a host of other problems.

Though massage therapists, physical therapists, and other soft tissue body workers can indirectly influence the spine with deep-tissue work on the tendons and ligaments, a misaligned and tight spine may require more direct attention. Osteopathic physicians who do manipulation (remember that not all do) and chiropractors are the two types of specialists most associated with manipulation of the spine itself. Just remember to avoid specialists who employ aggressive manipulation.

Common Treatment Reactions

Increased aches and pains: It's not at all unusual to experience increased aches, pains, or soreness in the body within the first 24 to 48 hours following a treatment, or even after starting a home stretching and exercising program. Sadly, this discomfort or even pain drives some people to discontinue treatments and home-exercise programs.

While it's understandable and prudent to be concerned about pain, more often than not the aches, pains, or soreness that follow a session are natural and unavoidable outcomes. The very act of introducing movement into a chronically tight and misaligned area of the body can cause temporary irritation and inflammation, or in other ways be aggravating to the body. This doesn't mean it isn't beneficial in the long run, however. I sometimes use the analogy of sweeping the attic: While it temporarily kicks up dust, which can be annoying, the attic will be much better off for it in the long run. The bottom line is that improving your alignment and reducing the tension in your body is a *process* and, although it will eventually be much happier, there are times when it will feel like a rocky course.

If you're concerned that you're being treated too aggressively or are stretching incorrectly, discuss your concerns with your practitioner, or ask someone knowledgeable to observe you as you stretch. Treatment reactions that do occur should diminish after each successive treatment or home session as the body gets looser and therefore more tolerant of the change being created. The quickest way to eliminate them is to be consistent in your efforts toward change, and to use the targeted movement, habit modification, and the advice of an outside practitioner on a regular basis.

Pops, clicks, and cracks: Also of concern to many of my middle- to older-aged patients are the "pops," "clicks," and "cracks" that they hear when they move, especially when they're exercising and doing range-of-motion maneuvers. The noises themselves are nothing more than the misaligned bones, tendons, and ligaments colliding with each other as they move. What concerns people is that these sounds often become more frequent and audible the more they exercise and the more they get treated by outside practitioners. The reason this happens is that as a result of utilizing the tools, the tension in the body is reduced, which creates more available movement, resulting in more of the body's structures bumping into each other. More than just harmless, this increase in sounds is a *good* sign, as it indicates that your body is getting looser. (If the body gets really loose, and better aligned, the sounds may begin to go away.)

CHAPTER NINE
Self-Treatment

The first duties of the physician is to educate the masses not to take medicine.

—Sir William Osler, MD

If you've ever been injured—or if you have a sports-loving child who's been injured—you're likely to be familiar with the RICE acronym. RICE stands for Rest, Ice, Compression, and Elevation, treatment strategies that are generally applied to sprains and strains that typically result in inflammation. (The signs of inflammation include redness, heat, swelling, pain, and compromised function.) Simply knowing the acronym is useful, but the more you understand about these four treatment strategies—and their sometimes more appropriate counterstrategies—the more effectively you'll be able to employ them. So let's take a closer look.

Rest versus Activity

Is it better to rest a body in pain or continue with activity? Well, that depends, in part, on the location of the pain and the reason for it. Pain and problems of the joints—the shoulders, elbows, hips, knees, and ankles—are the ones most frequently associated with inflammation and therefore benefit the most from rest. Without rest, the inflammation that results from moving injured areas can linger, causing scarring, destruction, and even the death of tissue. If you've ever tried it, however, you know that resting these areas can be a difficult task. It's hard to avoid using our arms and legs throughout the day, which is one of the reasons that pain and problems in these areas can linger for months.

Other areas of the body that frequently cause people pain include the neck, upper back, and lower back. Injuries and pain here are less often inflammatory and more often the result of muscle spasms and tension in the tendons and ligaments. Rather than rest, gentle activities like walking, stretching, and range-of-motion exercising tend to help these areas improve more quickly.

General Rest versus Activity Guidelines

1. Above all else, listen to your body. If it's telling you to stop all activity then do so. If it feels okay to move around (carefully, of course), then you should.

2. If you're injured and the injury has occurred within the past 48 hours, err on the side of rest. It's too easy to aggravate an injured area, thus prolonging recovery time.

If the pain or injury involves your lower back: I recommend that you lie on your back, on the floor, and then bend your knees and carefully raise up your lower legs, placing your calves on the seat of a chair or couch (figure 8-1). Resting in this position allows the lower back muscles to shorten and may help to decrease muscle spasms in the lower back area. Rest in this position for at least a minute and a half, but longer—even much longer—is fine as some people find this the most tolerable position to maintain when suffering from acute lower back pain. When

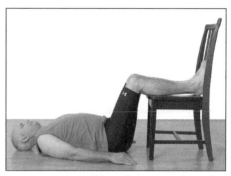

Figure 8-1

you're ready, roll to your side and get up *slowly*, using your arms rather than relying solely on your leg and back muscles.

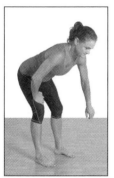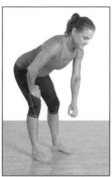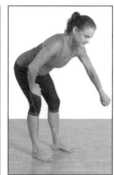

Figure 8-2

If the pain or injury involves your shoulder: Gentle arm circles are a good way to improve circulation and heal the area without stressing it. Lean forward from the hips, resting the weight of the upper body on your good arm, while letting the injured arm hang freely (figure 8-2). Using gravity, slowly begin doing clockwise circles with your arm, starting small and getting larger as you go. After 10 to 12 circles, let your arm gradually come to a stop, and then repeat the process going counterclockwise.

3. In addition to the above exercises, the stretches and range-of-motion exercises listed for each zone are safe and gentle and can be started early on in your recovery process. As with all things, however, "start low and go slow." In other words, proceed cautiously and stop if it hurts.

4. Strengthening should be attempted only after complete recovery from pain. Many patients with acute shoulder, lower back, or knee pain get re-injured doing strengthening activities using weights or Thera-Bands, often at the direction of a therapist. Strengthening exercises should be avoided until you are pain free. Gentle stretching movements and range-of-motion exercises are all that you should be doing beyond your normal daily activity.

5. It's never a good idea to take pain relievers, whether over-the-counter or prescription, as a way to more comfortably engage in physical activity. Pain relievers should be used strictly for pain relief. If you mute the pain and then go exercise, you risk doing more serious damage to your body. That's obviously not what you want!

Ice versus Heat

Whether to use ice or heat on a strained area is another question that can cause confusion. Not only does the answer rely on getting the correct diagnosis for one's pain but, to make matters worse, scientific researchers often debate what's actually going on within the body! As an example, the commonly used diagnosis of tendinitis—inflammation of the tendon—should, in many cases, be rediagnosed as tendinosis, as evidence often reveals few, if any, inflammatory cells are present.

That being said, when in doubt, icing should be the preferred choice. Cold inhibits circulation, which slows the inflammatory response. While it's true that inflammation is a normal reaction and part of the healing process, decreasing it in the early stages of an injury does appear to hasten recovery time.

General Guidelines

1. If you think your pain originates from a joint or the area right around it (like the shoulder, elbow, hip, knee, or ankle), use ice, as inflammation is likely involved. If it appears to be coming from a muscle, as pains in the neck, upper back, lower back, and buttock typically are, try heat. If you're not sure, use ice first and see how you feel, or alternate between the two.

2. If the area is red, warm, or swollen, or if you performed an activity that seems to have recently aggravated the area, causing an increase in pain, ice is probably the best choice.

3. Recent sprains, strains, and injuries—those that have occurred within 48 hours—should probably be treated with ice. Older aches and pains typically benefit more from heat, which promotes circulation and can relax muscles.

4. The best form of heat is wet, making showers, baths, warm washcloths, and hot water bottles great choices. Moist heat penetrates and soothes and, most importantly, loses its heat after a while. Heating pads are dry and stay warm, and can easily be overdone. Too much heat or heat applied too soon after a strain can make matters worse.

5. Never apply ice directly to the skin. Use a cloth the thickness of a T-shirt or dish towel to wrap the ice pack and apply until the skin is cold—approximately 15 minutes—then remove. Once the skin returns to room temperature, you can reapply the ice, repeating the process several times throughout the day.

Compression

Compression is used in the treatment of sprains and strains, and is usually achieved by wearing an ACE bandage or a brace on the injured area. The purpose of compression is to keep inflammation down and to ease pain by giving the involved joints and surrounding soft tissues support. The foot and ankle, the knee, and the lower back are the areas of the body on which compression is most frequently used.

While it's often appropriate to wear braces and support belts all the time during the acute phases of pain and injury, once that period is over, the role of compression becomes limited to guarding against re-injury. Wearing a knee brace when engaging in physical activities like hiking, playing tennis, or dancing at your child's wedding and wearing a lumbar belt to support the lower back when doing heavy physical labor are examples of using compression wisely to protect a vulnerable area. As a rule, however, you should not wear braces, belts, or other supports any longer than necessary. If you take the supporting job away from the local muscles and other soft tissues for too long, they'll eventually weaken, further destabilizing the area and preventing a full recovery.

Elevation

The purpose of elevating a body part is to slow the circulation of blood to it since blood has a harder time traveling uphill. Since blood brings pro-inflammatory components to an injured area, slowing the circulation is beneficial when fighting inflammation. Resting an inflamed knee or ankle on an ottoman is a typical application of the elevation concept. Whichever joint is injured, try to keep it resting at or above the level of the heart. Elevate the area as often as is convenient, until the swelling abates.

Joint Creams & Ointments

Many of my patients believe that they've experienced relief and quicker recovery from aches and pains by using one or more of the various muscle and joint creams, ointments, and gels that are on the market today. These topicals include such products as Tiger Balm, Biofreeze, Capsaicin, Topricin, Traumeel, and Arnica. All of these products are generally thought to be safe, and may go beyond pain relief to promote healing. Some feel cool when applied while others can feel quite hot. Just as their ingredients vary—from extract of hot peppers, to herbs, to homeopathic remedies—so do their mechanisms of action. If you feel so inclined, you might try one of these products and then take careful note of how you respond. Different people, as well as different injuries, will respond better to one than another.

Vitamin & Herbal Supplements

The world of vitamin and herbal supplements is large and growing every day. Modern science is regularly discovering new compounds, while older ones used by ancient civilizations are being rediscovered. Some of these civilizations have centuries of trial-and-error experience to draw on where the efficacy of their healing products is concerned. For instance, the Chinese have been using herbs, Indians have been using Ayurvedic compounds, and Native Americans have been using plant formulations for as long as there are records of their cultures.

There are many products on the market today that target joint and soft tissue health; some of them utilize wisdom from ancient cultures and traditions. The best of the non-pharmacological products provide relief to a sore muscle or inflamed joint and help in the body's repair process in a more natural way, and with fewer side effects, than prescription drugs and injections. The list below contains some of the products that I've used with my patients with good results.

It's important to note that when it comes to taking supplements, *quality counts*. Since the manufacturing process of supplements is loosely regulated, it's important to do a little homework and choose manufacturers who volunteer to have their products tested by third-party organizations. These organizations ensure that the products are consistently produced and controlled according to quality standards. The strictest standard is USP—United States Pharmacopeial Convention—and is available in some stores and is frequently sold by health-practitioners. GMP—Good Manufacturing Practice Regulations—is more readily available in stores and, though not nearly as strict, does give some assurance of quality.

CAUTION: Please consult an expert before starting a course of any of the following supplements, and under no circumstance take any herb or supplement without your doctor's approval if you're pregnant or nursing; take blood thinners or other medications; or have a serious medical condition.

For Acute Sprains, Strains, & Inflammation

- **Omega-3 fatty acids**: Possible anti-inflammatory effects used to alleviate stiffness and joint pain. EPA and DHA are primarily found in certain fish; ALA is found in plant sources such as nuts and seeds.

- **Boswellia serrata**: Commonly used in Ayurvedic medicine for osteoarthritis, rheumatoid arthritis, joint pain, bursitis, and tendinitis.

- **Bromelain**: Used as an anti-inflammatory for preventing muscle soreness after exercise; also used in conjunction with other ingredients in the treatment of arthritis. Bromelain is an enzyme found in pineapple juice and in the pineapple stem.

- **Tumeric (curcumin)**: Possible anti-inflammatory properties and is used to treat a wide variety of ailments, including arthritis. It's the main spice in curry.

- **MSM (methylsulfonylmethane)**: Possible anti-inflammatory properties, used for osteoarthritis, joint inflammation, rheumatoid arthritis, osteoporosis, bursitis, tendinitis, and muscle cramps. MSM is a chemical found in plants, animals, and humans.

- **Wobenzyme**: Possible anti-inflammatory properties used to treat osteoarthritis and to promote healing after injury. It's an enzyme preparation originally designed in Germany.

For Preventive Joint & Arthritis Support

- **Glucosamine sulfate**: Commonly used for osteoarthritis. It's a naturally occurring chemical found in the human body and is used in the production of tendons, ligaments, cartilage, and the fluid that surrounds joints.

- **Chondroitin sulfate**: May have some anti-inflammatory properties and is used to improve joint function and slow the progression of osteoarthritis. It's a component of human connective tissues and is found in cartilage and bone. In supplements, chondroitin sulfate is usually derived from animal cartilage. Often packaged together with glucosamine sulfate.

- **Omega-3 fatty acids**: Possible anti-inflammatory effects used to alleviate stiffness and joint pain. EPA and DHA are primarily found in certain fish; ALA is found in plant sources such as nuts and seeds.

- **Hyaluronic acid**: Used for various joint disorders, including osteoarthritis, by acting as a cushion and lubricant. It can be taken by mouth or injected into the affected joint. Hyaluronic acid is a substance that's naturally present in the human body; the highest concentrations are in the fluids of the eyes and joints.

- **MSM (methylsulfonylmethane)**: Possible anti-inflammatory properties, used for osteoarthritis, joint inflammation, rheumatoid arthritis, osteoporosis, bursitis, tendinitis, and muscle cramps. MSM is a chemical found in plants, animals, and humans.

- **Turmeric (curcumin)**: Possible anti-inflammatory properties and is used to treat a wide variety of ailments, including arthritis. It's the main spice in curry.

- **Wobenzyme**: Possible anti-inflammatory properties used to treat osteoarthritis and to promote healing after injury. It's an enzyme preparation originally designed in Germany.

You can frequently find the individual ingredients listed above packaged together, labeled, and sold as anti-arthritis formulations, joint pain-relief products, or anti-inflammatory formulas to treat strains and sprains.

Painkillers & Anti-Inflammatories

Pharmaceutical drugs have important roles to play in many healing processes. Painkillers and anti-inflammatories, for instance, can be lifesavers in certain situations. But it's critical to understand that pharmaceuticals should have limited use in the care of the human frame.

Unlike vitamin and herbal supplements, pharmaceutical drugs do very little to assist in the actual *repair* process of the musculoskeletal system. Rather, they're designed to treat symptoms, and they do so with often harmful side effects. In addition, pharmaceutical pain-relieving drugs can mute pain so effectively that you run the risk of sustaining further damage to the body, as without pain you may feel free to continue activities that are worsening your condition! It's similar to responding to a knocking sound coming from your car's engine by wearing a pair of ear plugs; if you can't hear the trouble, you may continue to do damage and wind up down the road completely out of commission. For all of these reasons, drugs designed to address pain and inflammation should not be the main focus in the treatment of the musculoskeletal system and should be used sparingly, if at all.

NSAIDs

Over-the-counter non-steroidal anti-inflammatories (NSAIDs), like ibuprofen (Advil) and naproxen (Aleve), are generally effective at reducing the mild to moderate pain and inflammation from acute sprains and strains. They're preferable to the stronger narcotic painkillers (Vicodin, Percocet), which have worse side effects and can mute pain so much that you have even less chance to hear your body's signals. In the short term, NSAIDs can be used for sprains and strains, but I don't recommend them for long-term use. They do nothing to help the body's repair process, and have been shown to increase the risk of such things as heart attacks, strokes, liver and kidney damage, and possibly to inhibit cartilage repair and accelerate bone loss.

Muscle Relaxants

Muscle relaxants (Soma, Flexeril, Skelaxin, Robaxin), which are frequently prescribed by physicians for muscle pain, should probably be renamed "brain relaxants" because they generally work in the brain as sedatives. Their mechanism of action is to make you too dopey to do anything but rest, which may actually be useful for some people, especially those who are in pain but have a hard time slowing down and relaxing. As you may or may not know, your respiratory diaphragm, that very important structure that allows you to breath, is itself a muscle. If muscle relaxers really relaxed *muscles*, you'd stop breathing! Side effects for this class of drugs include drowsiness, seizures, urinary retention, irregular heartbeat, and possible addiction. I see few reasons to take these medications, and many not to take them.

Cortisone & Anesthetic Injections

Physicians use various injections into the joints, spine, and surrounding tissues (where the tendons and bursa live) to address musculoskeletal pain. The goal is generally to decrease pain and/or inflammation for immediate relief, or to assist in the rehabilitation process (patients may participate more in rehabilitation exercises when they have less pain). As with oral medications, however, the problem with this approach is the focus it places on the symptoms and, in this case, the side effects from a needle stuck in your body and noxious chemicals injected. Side effects include possible damage to nearby bone, nerve damage, tendon rupture, and deterioration of joint cartilage—which limits the number of shots into a joint that you can receive.

Inversion & Traction

Inverting the body or using traction—a pulling force—are methods of attempting to decompress the muscles, joints, spine, and discs of the body in order to counter the effects of trauma or gravity. The idea that decompression is beneficial has a certain logic to it, but it's somewhat controversial all the same. Some say that decompressing the body and defying gravity is impossible because the body is too tightly held together with tendons, ligaments, and muscles and won't budge a millimeter without the use of severe force (and by now you know that I don't advocate severe force). Others swear by it and can cite this recent study:

> A 2012 study was performed at the neurosurgery department of James Cook University in the United Kingdom on patients with back pain and sciatica who had documented lumbar protuberant disc disease and were awaiting surgery. It concluded that "intermittent traction with an inversion device resulted in significant reduction in the need for surgery."[33]

Personally, I'd only recommend the inversion method where you get strapped to a chair or table and tilted about 30 degrees short of completely upside down, letting gravity and the weight of the body do the work. I'd never recommend any form of traction where an outside force, such as the over-the-door weighted contraption designed for the neck, is involved. That's just asking for trouble. If you decide to try a tilt chair or table, start slowly and be sure to have a spotter with you—someone to make sure no accidents happen. I recommend that you consult your physician first, and definitely avoid inversion if you suffer from a heart condition, have glaucoma or a retinal detachment, or are pregnant.

Massage Ball/Foam Roller Treatment

Several of my patients have discovered that painful areas of the body can be relieved through a sort of self-massage using a rubber ball, foam roller, or similar device. (One patient discovered that using one of her cat's toys worked well!) The idea is to lie on the floor or stand against a wall and position a soft, spongy ball or other similar item in such a way that you can roll around on it until it hits a tender area, which is likely a muscle "knot." Then, pushing with your body, put a little gentle pressure into the ball and massage the area (figure 8-3).

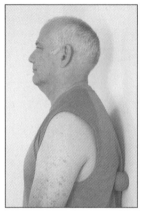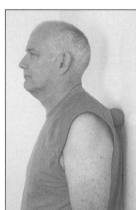

Figure 8-3

This self-massage technique can be tried anywhere on the body but is especially effective for neck pain that comes from the muscles of the upper neck or base of the skull (*suboccipitals*); upper back pain, in particular the area between the shoulder blades that's hard for people to reach themselves (*rhomboids*); and butt pain, the kind that's right in the fleshy part of the muscle (*piriformis*). Foam rollers can also work well for the butt muscles, as well as for the larger muscles and broader parts of the body—like the lower and upper back, arms, and legs.

Whichever method you choose, be careful not to overdo the massage, even though it might feel good. Too much pressure could potentially irritate a muscle or inflame a joint.

Leaning into a Corner— Self-Treatment for Zone 1

This is a very useful technique for alleviating upper back and sometimes neck pain, and all it requires is your body and two walls that meet at a 90-degree angle. Many of my patients swear by this technique, especially for addressing the stabbing-type pain that occurs between the shoulder blades.

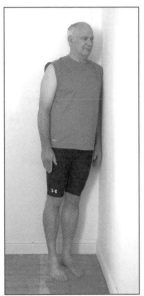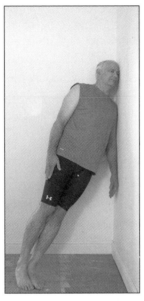

1. Stand in the corner of a room and place your shoulder so that it's sandwiched between the walls.

2. Now, while leaving your shoulder pressed into the corner, walk your feet away from the corner (your feet will be moving on a line that bisects the angle of the corner, and your shoulder will slide down a little bit) so that you're leaning your body—using all of your body weight—into the corner through your shoulder. The shoulder in the corner should be the one on the same side as the upper back or neck pain. If you're not sure which side is more painful, or if the pain is in the middle, do both sides.

By leaning into the corner, the shoulder gets pressed in toward the body, moving the shoulder blade on that side—which through rounding has undoubtedly migrated away from the spine—closer to the spine. Temporarily moving the shoulder back where it belongs both shortens and relaxes the tight upper back muscles *(rhomboids)* and the muscle that connects the shoulder, upper back, and neck *(trapezius)*, which are frequently in spasm and causing pain.

Make sure to hold this leaning position for a minimum of 90 seconds before you return to your normal standing position in order to allow the muscles to fully relax. If it worked, you'll feel better almost immediately. If not, you can try repeating the process on the other side.

Walk Barefoot on the Earth— Self-Treatment for Zone 3

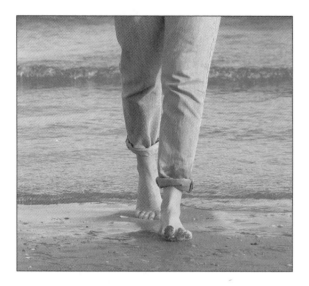

Walking barefoot outside is a great way to exercise the muscles and other soft tissues of the feet that have become weaker over time due to being stuck in shoes all day long. While walking barefoot around the house does offer some exercise for the feet, it's not ideal. The hard surfaces of our wood, tile, concrete, and synthetic floors don't support the arches of the feet and don't work the muscles as hard as walking outside on the earth does. Whether on grass, soil, or sand (the best workout), the softer and more yielding surfaces of the earth will simultaneously cushion the feet and force the individual muscles to become more engaged as they work harder to propel you forward—doing the work they were designed to do. Weather and locale permitting (be careful in public parks), I recommend you try to do some outdoor barefoot walking daily.

While this self-treatment focuses on the feet, it has the added benefit of exercising all of the muscles of the legs. Moreover, because the feet are the foundations of the body, walking barefoot outdoors can positively influence the whole musculoskeletal system.

CHAPTER TEN
Moving Forward: Two Steps to Keeping Healthy

We do not stop exercising because we grow old—
we grow old because we stop exercising.

—Dr. Kenneth Cooper

As we reach middle age, our bodies begin to decline slowly but steadily, becoming tighter, more misaligned, and weaker. That's the bad news. The good news is that we can dramatically slow down this process. We can release tension from our frames, improve our alignment, and get stronger. The choice is simple: We can either actively move toward health or, by default, move farther away from it. If health is your goal, these two steps will help.

Step 1: Use Your Toolbox

Maintaining a grip-free body is as simple as utilizing the Hammer (page 14), the Crowbar (page 87), and the Carpenter (page 98) on a regular basis. Don't make the common mistake of waiting until something hurts before grabbing a tool and taking action. You should do the stretches and range-of-motion exercises *daily*, the strengthening exercises *three times a week*, pay attention to your modern living habits *regularly*, and get treatments by outside practitioners *routinely* for maintenance and prevention. If you wait until you're in pain, some damage may already have been done or, at the very least, healing will take longer and require more effort.

Following are some tips to help you be consistent with your tools and enjoy a pain-free body that supports you in all of your life's endeavors.

Tips on Stretches, Strengthening, & Range-of-Motion Exercises

- Make copies of the exercises and post them on the walls or mirrors in several areas where you can see them. *In Sight = In Mind*.

- The best time to stretch is *now*. It doesn't matter what time of the day you do the exercises, what's important is that you do them. In fact, if you're creative, you can work in your stretches and range-of-motion exercises while waiting in line at the store, sitting at the doctor's office, or talking on the phone.

Tips on Modern Living Modifications

- Install a computer program that reminds you to take a break every 20 minutes while you're sitting at your desk.

- Post reminders at your desk to sit up straight, take breaks, move your arms and shoulders, and uncross your legs.

- Buy some accessories. Accessories can not only help you to break the grip but can also be fun to use and are visual reminders to get active.

  - a foam roller or sponge balls for self-massage

  - a foam bolster to perform the shoulder and chest stretch

  - a book stand for reading for better head posture

  - shoe gel inserts to cushion the feet

  - a body pillow for sleeping

  - a wedge pillow to sit on to improve your posture

Visit my website endeverydaypain.com for more ideas and information.

Tips on the Use of the Outside Practitioner

- Talk to friends, relatives, or acquaintances about positive experiences they've had with outside practitioners.

- Set some money aside every month to be used for hands-on maintenance treatments.

Step 2: Know Your Why

In order to take consistent action to break the grip on your body, you must know exactly why you're doing it. Old habits can be hard to break and new ones hard to make unless doing so has real meaning for you. *While pain relief is a great motivator, it will need to be replaced by other reasons once the pain goes away.* Some positive motivating reasons I've heard from my patients include: to be able to play catch with a grandchild in ten years; to be able to dance at a 50th wedding anniversary party or at a child or grandchild's wedding; to continue to enjoy golf, travel, or tending a garden well into one's 70s, 80s, and 90s.

Here are a few tips to help you stay motivated and create lasting good habits:

- Visualize a life where your body does not get in the way of your living it fully.

- Recite the mantra "Use it or lose it!" It's up to you.

- Create some dedicated self-improvement time. Get up 15 minutes earlier every day to stretch and exercise. It will change your life!

And, remember, breaking the grip of long-term molding on your body will not only benefit your joints and muscles, keeping you active for as long as you'd like, but it will also benefit the nerves, arteries, and organs that live within the musculoskeletal system—keeping you healthier while you're here!

A Word about Aerobic Exercise

No book about the care of the human body would be complete without a discussion of aerobic exercise, and I've saved that discussion until now for a very important reason. Breaking the grip in order to create more space in the body, the ultimate goal of this book, is essential not only in the prevention and cure of chronic aches and pains, it also plays a vital role in preparing the body for the demands of an aerobic exercise routine.

As previously mentioned, I've known scores of middle-aged and older patients who, at the request of a doctor or loved ones, embarked on an aerobic exercise program only to be quickly sidelined due to pain in the knees, hips, or elsewhere. My recommendation, therefore, is that you use the tools presented in this book for at least four to six weeks before beginning a new routine of physical exercise, or before returning to an old one that you were forced to abandon. Your stronger, looser body will thank you.

Once you're armed with a body better prepared to handle it, I strongly recommend that you begin a regular routine of at least moderate physical exercise. It would take another book to describe all of the known benefits of aerobic exercise, so let's just list a few of them and then agree that aerobic exercise is crucial to the health and well-being of your body and mind. Aerobic exercise:

- Strengthens the heart, reducing blood pressure, heart disease, and other cardiovascular problems

- Promotes circulation, providing life-giving oxygen to the body

- Increases lymphatic drainage for more efficient removal of waste from the body

- Lubricates joints, thereby decreasing friction, wear, and tear

- Keeps muscles and other soft tissues flexible and pliable

- Increases metabolism, helping to keep weight down

- Supports the mind, boosting mood, memory, and the sense of well-being

- Improves balance, helping to reduce falls and injury

- Increases stamina and boosts energy while also promoting sound sleep

What more encouragement do you need?

Moderate aerobic exercise is described as approximately 30 minutes of continuous movement causing you to be slightly out of breath, meaning that you're able to talk but not effortlessly. It usually involves brief warm-up and cool-down periods. Typical moderate aerobic activities include swimming, walking briskly, hiking moderately challenging terrain, and biking roads that contain some hills. Recommendations change, and while it appears that even 10 minutes of exercise is beneficial, 30 minutes of continuous activity performed three or more times a week is the current recommended goal. Curiously, there's some evidence that more than 30 minutes may be detrimental! And remember: Check with your doctor to get clearance before you begin any aerobic conditioning routine.

Mix It Up—Cross Training

Depending on your condition and any specific challenges, you should try to include a variety of different activities in your exercise routine. Walking one day a week, swimming a second day, and bicycling on a third day will ensure that you keep lots of muscles strong and healthy, and mixing it up means less repetitive wear and tear on the joints. Or you might try running, playing basketball, and rowing, or hiking, tennis, and an elliptical machine. Too many people create or worsen shoulder, lower back, hip, knee, or foot pain through the routine repetition of just one form of exercise.

NOTE: If you're prone to hip, knee, or foot pain and problems, give the break-the-grip exercises longer to work, and then choose aerobic activities that are primarily non-weight bearing. Examples of non-weight bearing exercises include swimming, rowing, and bicycling.

Just Do It!

When it comes to the care of the human frame, moving toward health doesn't have to be time consuming or complicated, but it does have to be done. As you now know after reading this book, without preventive measures, the middle-aged and older body becomes gripped and molded, leading to misalignment and tension, a succession of muscle and joint pains, and repeated medical and surgical interventions. Fortunately, armed with the knowledge in this book, you now have the tools to cure and prevent this breakdown of the body.

And the tools work. I've seen the results with many of my patients. One such patient, a man in his late 50s, came to my office with a complaint of lower back pain and sciatica—pain radiating down his right leg—that his orthopedist informed him was due to a herniated disc. Although surgery had been recommended, he decided to seek an alternative and was referred to me. Though it took a couple of months, a combination of gentle hands-on work, daily lower back stretches, and eventually strengthening exercises resolved his problem and he was able to avoid surgery.

It's important to understand that results don't always come quickly—an over-50-year-old body has often accumulated a lot of stress, strain, and bad habits—but a little daily effort can have a major impact and get the body turned around and moving in the right direction. Recall what the newfound daily habit of brushing and flossing did for the health of the teeth and gums! The end result is a life with less pain and fewer problems, and a body that supports you in all of your endeavors.

I wish you health and success!

Endnotes

1. J. E. Bible, D. Biswas, C. P. Miller, P. G. Whang, J. N. Grauer, "Normal functioning range of motion of the cervical spine during 15 activities of daily living," *Journal of Spinal Disorders & Techniques* (2010): 15–21.

2. G. Bronfort, N. Nilsson, M. Haas, R. Evans, C. H. Goldsmith, W. J. Assendfelt, L. M. Bouter, "Non-invasive physical treatments for chronic/recurrent headache," *Cochrane Database of Systematic Reviews* 3 (2004): CD001878. Wolfe-Harris Center for Clinical Studies, Northwestern Health Sciences University, Bloomington, MN.

3. G. Bronfort, W. J. Assendelft, R. Evans, M. Haas, L. Bouter, "Efficacy of spinal manipulation for chronic headache: a systematic review," *Journal of Manipulative and Physiological Therapeutics* 24, no. 7 (September 2001): 457–66.

4. S. D. Boden, P. R. McCowin, D. O. Davis, T. S. Dina, A. S. Mark, S. Wiesel, "Abnormal magnetic-resonance scans of the cervical spine in asymptomatic subjects. A prospective investigation," *Journal of Bone and Joint Surgery. American Volume* 72, no. 8 (September 1990): 1178–84.

5. T. M. Kay, A. Gross, C. Goldsmith, P. L. Santaguida, J. Hoving, G. Bronfort, "Exercises for mechanical neck disorders," *Cochrane Database of Systematic Reviews* 3 (July 20, 2005): CD004250. Physiotherapy Services, Sunnybrook & Women's College Health Sciences Centre, North York, ON, Canada.

6. E. Solem-Bertoft, K. A. Thuomas, C. E. Westerberg, "The influence of scapular retraction and protraction on the width of the subacromial space: An MRI study," *Clinical Orthopaedics and Related Research* 296 (November 1993): 99–103.

7. S. Gumina, G. Di Giorgio, F. Postacchini, "Subacromial space in adult patients with thoracic hyperkyphosis and in healthy volunteers," *La Chirurgia degli Organi di Movimento* 91, no. 2 (February 2008): 93–96.

8. J. E. Kuhn, "Exercise in the treatment of rotator cuff impingement: a systematic review and a synthesized evidence-based rehabilitation protocol," *Journal of Shoulder and Elbow Surgery* 18, no. 1 (January–February 2009): 138–60.

9. J. A. Coghlan, R. Buchbinder, S. Green, R. V. Johnson, S. N. Bell, "Surgery for rotator cuff disease," *Cochrane Database of Systematic Reviews* 1 (January 23, 2008): CD005619.

10. J. E. Kuhn, "Exercise in the treatment of rotator cuff impingement: a systematic review and a synthesized evidence-based rehabilitation protocol," *Journal of Shoulder and Elbow Surgery* 18, no. 1 (January–February 2009): 138–60.

11. G. Senbursa, G. Baltaci, O. A. Atay, "The effectiveness of manual therapy in supraspinatus tendinopathy," *Acta Orthopaedica et Traumatologica Turcica* 45, no. 3 (2011): 162–67.

12. M. J. Willemink, H. W. Van Es, P. H. Helmhout, A. L. Diederik, J. C. Kelder, J. P. van Heesewijk, "The effects of dynamic isolated lumbar extensor training on lumbar multifidus functional cross-sectional area and functional status of patients with chronic non-specific low back pain," *Spine* 37, no. 26 (December 15, 2012): E1651–58.

13. A. G. Filler, J. Haynes, S. E. Jordan, et al., "Sciatica of nondisc origin and piriformis syndrome: diagnosis by magnetic resonance neurography and interventional magnetic resonance imaging with outcome study of resulting treatment," *Journal of Neurosurgery: Spine* 2, no. 2 (February 2005): 99–115.

14. W. C. Jacobs, M. van Tulder, M. Arts, et al., "Surgery versus conservative management of sciatica due to a lumbar herniated disc: a systematic review," *European Spine Journal* 20, no. 4 (April 2011): 513–22.

15. M. Jensen, M. Brant-Zawadzki, et al., "Magnetic resonance imaging of the lumbar spine in people without back pain," *The New England Journal of Medicine* 331, no. 2 (July 14, 1994): 69–73.

16. A. J. Haig, M. E. Geisser, et al., "Electromyographic and magnetic resonance imaging to predict lumbar stenosis, low-back pain, and no back symptoms," *Journal of Bone and Joint Surgery. American Volume* 89, no. 2 (February 2007): 358–66.

17. S. D. Boden, D. O. Davis, T. S. Dina, N. J. Patronas, S. W. Wiesel, "Abnormal magnetic-resonance scans of the lumbar spine in asymptomatic subjects: A prospective investigation," *Journal of Bone and Joint Surgery. American Volume* 72, no. 3 (March 1990): 403–408.

18. A. J. Haig, M. E. Geisser, et al. ""Electromyographic and magnetic resonance imaging to predict lumbar stenosis, low-back pain, and no back symptoms," *Journal of Bone and Joint Surgery. American Volume* 89, no. 2 (February 2007): 358–66.

19. CBSNews.com, "A New Hope for Back Pain Sufferers?," May 6, 2012. www.cbsnews.com/8301-3445_162-57428677/a-new-hope-for-back-pain-sufferers.

20. J. I. Brox, R. Sorensen, A. Friis, et al., "Randomized clinical trial of lumbar instrumented fusion and cognitive intervention and exercises in patients with chronic low back pain and disc degeneration," *Spine* 28, no. 17 (September 1, 2003): 1913–21.

21. J. Fairbank, H. Frost, J. Wilson-MacDonald, L. M. Yu, K. Barker, R. Collins, "Randomised controlled trial to compare surgical stabilisation of the lumbar spine with an intensive rehabilitation programme for patients with chronic low back pain: the MRC spine stabilisation trial," *BMJ* 330, no. 7502 (May 28, 2005): 1233.

22. A. D. Beswick, V. Wylde, R. Gooberman-Hill, A. Blom, P. Dieppe, "What proportion of patients report long-term pain after total hip or knee replacement for osteoarthritis? A systematic review of prospective studies in unselected patients," *BMJ Open* 2, no. 1 (February 22, 2012): e000435.

23. B. Register, A. T. Pennock, et al., "Prevalence of abnormal hip findings in asymptomatic participants: a prospective, blinded study," *The American Journal of Sports Medicine* 40, no. 12 (2012): 2720–24.

24. D. G. Blakenbaker, S. R. Ullrick, et al. "Correlation of MRI findings with clinical findings of trochanteric pain syndrome," *Skeletal Radiology* 37, no. 10 (October 2008): 903–909.

25. T. Bhattacharyya, D. Gale, P. Dewire, et al., "The clinical importance of meniscal tears demonstrated by magnetic resonance imaging in osteoarthritis of the knee," *Journal of Bone and Joint Surgery. American Volume* 85-A, no. 1 (October 2008): 4–9.

26. M. T. Hannan, D. T. Felson, T. Pincus, "Analysis of the discordance between radiographic changes and knee pain in osteoarthritis of the knee," *Journal of Rheumatology* 27, no. 6 (June 2006): 1513–17.

27. J. Bedson, P. R. Croft, "The discordance between clinical and radiographic knee osteoarthritis: a systematic search and summary of the literature," *BMC Musculoskeletal Disorders* 9 (September 2, 2008): 116.

28. M. T. Hannan, D. T. Felson, T. Pincus, "Analysis of the discordance between radiographic changes and knee pain in osteoarthritis of the knee," *Journal of Rheumatology* 27, no. 6 (June 2006): 1513–17.

29. D. Hunt, H. Prather, M. Harris, J. C. Clohisy, "Clinical outcomes analysis of conservative and surgical treatment of patients with clinical indications of prearthritic, intra-articular hip disorders," *PM&R* 4, no. 7 (July 2012): 479–87.

30. S. Herrlin, M. Hallander, et al., "Arthroscopic or conservative treatment of degenerative medial meniscus tears: a prospective randomized trial," *Knee Surgery, Sports Traumatology, Arthroscopy* 15, no. 4 (April 2007): 393–401.

31. J. E. Kuhn. "Exercise in the treatment of rotator cuff impingement: a systematic review and a synthesized evidence-based rehabilitation protocol," *Journal of Shoulder and Elbow Surgery* 18, no. 1 (January–February 2009): 138–60.

32. G. Senbursa, G. Baltaci, O. A. Atay, "The effectiveness of manual therapy in supraspinatus tendinopathy," *Acta Orthopaedica et Traumatologica Turcica* 45, no. 3 (2011): 162–67.

33. K. S. Prasad, B. A. Gregson, G. Hargreaves, T. Byrnes, P. Winburn, A. D. Mendelow, "Inversion therapy in patients with pure single level lumbar discogenic disease: a pilot randomized trial," *Disability and Rehabilitation* 34, no. 17 (2012): 1473–80.

Resources

Alter, Judy. *Stretch & Strengthen*. Boston: Houghton Mifflin, 1986.

Carey, Anthony B. *The Pain-Free Program: A Proven Method to Relieve Back, Neck, Shoulder, and Joint Pain*. Hoboken, NJ: John Wiley & Sons, 2005.

Chew, Ming, and Stephanie Golden. *The Permanent Pain Cure: The Breakthrough Way to Heal Your Muscle and Joint Pain for Good*. New York: McGraw Hill, 2008.

DeStefano, Rob, and Bryan Kelly. *Muscle Medicine: The Revolutionary Approach to Maintaining, Strengthening, and Repairing Your Muscles and Joints*. New York: Fireside, 2009.

Dimon, Theodore Jr. *The Body in Motion: Its Evolution and Design*. Berkeley, CA: North Atlantic Books, 2011.

DiNubile, Nicholas A. *FrameWork: Your 7-Step Program for Healthy Muscles, Bones, and Joints*. New York: Rodale, 2005.

Egoscue, Pete, and Roger Gittines. *Pain Free: A Revolutionary Method for Stopping Chronic Pain*. New York: Bantam Books, 1998.

Gokhale, Esther, and Susan Adams. *8 Steps to a Pain-Free Back: Natural Posture Solutions for Pain in the Back, Neck, Shoulder, Hip, Knee, and Foot*. California: Pendo Press, 2008.

Goodman, Eric, and Peter Park. *Foundation: Redefine Your Core, Conquer Back Pain, and Move with Confidence*. New York: Rodale, 2011.

Johnson, Jim. *Treat Your Own Knee Arthritis*. Indianapolis, IN: Dog Ear Publishing, 2011.

Johnson, Jim. *Treat Your Own Rotator Cuff*. Indianapolis, IN: Dog Ear Publishing, 2006.

Johnson, Jim. *Treat Your Own Spinal Stenosis*. Indianapolis, IN: Dog Ear Publishing, 2010.

McKenzie, Robin, and Craig Kubey. *7 Steps to a Pain-Free Life: How to Rapidly Relieve Back, Neck, and Shoulder Pain*. New York: Plume, 2000.

Metzl, Jordan D., and Andrew Heffernan. *The Exercise Cure: A Doctor's All-Natural, No-Pill Prescription for Better Health and Longer Life*. New York: Rodale, 2013.

Murray, Michael T. *Encyclopedia of Nutritional Supplements: The Essential Guide for Improving Your Health Naturally*. Roseville, CA: Prima Publishing, 1996.

Porter, Kathleen. *Ageless Spine, Lasting Health: The Open Secret to Pain-Free Living and Comfortable Aging*. Austin, TX: Synergy Books, 2006.

Schatz, Bernard. *Chronic Pain! The Overlooked Simplicity*. Ruckersville, VA: Ascara Publishing Company, 2013.

Still, A. T. *Osteopathy Research & Practice*. Seattle: Eastland Press, 1992.

Weisberg, Joseph, and Heidi Shink. *3 Minutes to a Pain-Free Life: The Groundbreaking Program for Total Body Pain Prevention and Rapid Relief*. New York: Atria Books, 2005.

Wharton, Jim, and Phil Wharton. *The Whartons' Stretch Book*. New York: Times Books, 1996.

Index

Acknowledgments

I once heard that writers don't write because they can, but because they're willing to. And while it's true that I was willing, I couldn't have done it without a lot of other people making it possible.

Special thanks to my editor Nan Gatewood Satter, who not only made my writing better but also skillfully put the material into a more meaningful sequence. A big thanks to Casie Vogel, acquisitions editor at Ulysses Press, who enthusiastically recognized the value of my book, and to Jake Flaherty and all of the other talented people at Ulysses for making it a reality. I am also grateful to the osteopathic physicians who shared their passion for healing and their love of osteopathy through their teachings, especially Hugh Ettlinger, DO, Jim Jealous, DO, and Jeff Greenfield, DO. A profound thanks to all of my patients who entrusted me with their care. To quote Dr. Andrew Taylor Still, "I see God in their faces and forms."

And, most importantly, thanks to my loving and supportive family. To my wife Janice, my partner in life who believed in me as an author before I did. If it wasn't for her support and encouragement, this book would not be possible. To my daughter Alexis, who constantly reminds me to live in the moment and gives me joy on a daily basis. To my mom, who taught me to be passionate about life and love what you do. To my dad, who instilled in me the value of hard work; he would've loved to have seen this book completed. And to the rest of my family, who all have helped me to become the person I am, whose life is dedicated to helping others.

About the Author

Dr. Joseph Tieri is an osteopathic medical physician and a specialist in the holistic hands-on healing practice of osteopathic manipulation. He has been in private practice for more than 16 years and has treated thousands of adults and children suffering from a variety of ailments. Dr. Tieri has lectured and published articles on alternative medicine and osteopathy and serves as a clinical instructor teaching medical students and residents at his office, the Stone Ridge Healing Arts Center in Stone Ridge, New York, of which he is part owner. He enjoys raising his daughter Alexis with his wife Janice, and his hobbies include hiking and skiing in the Catskill Mountains and practicing karate, in which he holds a black-belt degree. For more information and resources to assist you in your quest to end everyday pain, please visit his website, EndEverydayPain.com.